T0186120

Register Now for Online Access to Your Book!

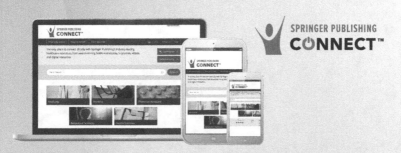

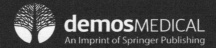

demosMEDICAL
An Imprint of Springer Publishing

View all our products at springerpub.com/demosmedical

Practical Guide to Botulinum Toxin Injections

Surendra Barshikar, MD
Fatma Gul, MD, MSc
Merrine Klakeel, DO
Amy Mathews, MD

Illustrations by
Shashank B. Karvekar, MBBS, DNB

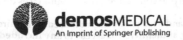

demosMEDICAL
An Imprint of Springer Publishing

Springer Publishing Company, LLC
11 West 42nd Street, New York, NY 10036
www.springerpub.com
connect.springerpub.com/

Acquisitions Editor: Beth Barry
Compositor: S4Carlisle Publishing Services

ISBN: 978-0-8261-4868-1
ebook ISBN: 978-0-8261-4869-8
DOI: 10.1891/9780826148698

20 21 22 23 24 / 5 4 3 2 1

Medicine is an ever-changing science. Research and clinical experience are continually
expanding our knowledge , in particular our understanding of proper treatment and
drug therapy. The authors, editors, and publisher have made every effort to ensure
that all information in this book is in accordance with the state of knowledge at the
time of production of the book. Nevertheless, the authors, editors, and publisher are
not responsible for any errors or omissions or for any consequence from application
of the information in this book and make no warranty, expressed or implied, with
respect to the content of this publication. Every reader should examine carefully the
package inserts accompanying each drug and should carefully check whether the
dosage schedules therein or the contraindications stated by the manufacturer differ
from the statements made in this book. Such examination is particularly important
with drugs that are either rarely used or have been newly released on the market.

Library of Congress Cataloging-in-Publication Data

Names: Barshikar, Surendra, editor. | Gul, Fatma, editor. | Klakeel,
    Merrine, editor. | Mathews, Amy, editor.
Title: Practical guide to botulinum toxin injections / [edited by] Surendra
    Barshikar, MD, Fatma Gul, MD, MSc, Merrine Klakeel, DO, Amy Mathews, MD ;
    illustrations by Shashank B. Karvekar, MBBS, DNB.
Description: New York : Springer Publishing Company, 2021. | Includes
    bibliographical references and index.
Identifiers: LCCN 2020049195 (print) | LCCN 2020049196 (ebook) | ISBN
    9780826148681 (cloth) | ISBN 9780826148698 (ebook)
Subjects: LCSH: Botulinum toxin. | Botulinum toxin–Therapeutic use.
Classification: LCC RC935.S64 P72 2021 (print) | LCC RC935.S64 (ebook) |
    DDC 615.3/29364–dc23
LC record available at https://lccn.loc.gov/2020049195
LC ebook record available at https://lccn.loc.gov/2020049196

Contact sales@springerpub.com to receive discount rates on bulk purchases.

Publisher's Note: **New and used products purchased from third-party sellers are not
guaranteed for quality, authenticity, or access to any included digital components.**

Printed in the United States of America.

Contents

Part I. Introduction

Part II. Clinical Applications: Upper Limb Spasticity and Dystonia

Part III. Clinical Applications: Lower Limb Spasticity and Dystonia

Part IV. Clinical Applications: Axial Spasticity and Dystonia

Part V. Other Clinical Applications

Part VI. Clinical Syndromes

Contributors

AUTHORS

Surendra Barshikar, MD
Assistant Professor
Department of Physical Medicine and Rehabilitation Medicine
University of Texas Southwestern Medical Center
Dallas, Texas

Fatma Gul, MD, MSc
Professor
Department of Physical Medicine and Rehabilitation Medicine
University of Texas Southwestern Medical Center
Dallas, Texas

Merrine Klakeel, DO
Assistant Professor
Department of Physical Medicine and Rehabilitation Medicine
University of Texas Southwestern Medical Center
Dallas, Texas

Amy Mathews, MD
Assistant Professor
Department of Physical Medicine and Rehabilitation Medicine
University of Texas Southwestern Medical Center
Dallas, Texas

ILLUSTRATOR

Shashank B. Karvekar, MBBS, DNB
Director
Chief Orthopedic Surgeon
Karvekar Hospital
Consultant Orthopedic Surgeon
Markandeya Hospital
Solapur, India

CONTRIBUTORS

Shilpa Chitnis, MD, PhD, FAAN, DANA
Professor
Department of Neurology and Neurotherapeutics
University of Texas Southwestern Medical Center
Dallas, Texas
Chapter 16. Blepharospasm

Mazen Elkurd, DO
Instructor
Department of Neurology and Neurotherapeutics
University of Texas Southwestern Medical Center
Dallas, Texas
Chapter 14. Cervical Dystonia

Rasheda El-Nazer, MD
Movement Disorders Fellow
Department of Neurology and Neurotherapeutics
University of Texas Southwestern Medical Center
Dallas, Texas
Chapter 16. Blepharospasm

Ramy S. Goueli, MD, MHS
Female Pelvic Medicine and Reconstructive Urology Fellow
Department of Urology
University of Texas Southwestern Medical Center
Dallas, Texas
Chapter 19. Chemodenervation of the Lower Urinary Tract

Kamel Itani, MD
Professor
Department of Ophthalmology
University of Texas Southwestern Medical Center
Dallas, Texas
Chapter 20. Glabellar Rhytides

Gary E. Lemack, MD
Professor of Urology and Neurology
Rose Mary Haggar Professor of Urology
Residency Program Director in Urology
University of Texas Southwestern Medical Center
Dallas, Texas
Chapter 19. Chemodenervation of the Lower Urinary Tract

Foreword

What a pleasure it is to write a foreword to *Practical Guide to Botulinum Toxin Injections*. During my first decade of physiatric practice, my tools for addressing spasticity and muscle hypertonicity were limited to casting/splinting, phenol injections, and surgery. The availability of neurotoxins has truly altered the approach to the management of spasticity (as well as bestowing youthfulness upon many a brow that previously was furrowed). While phenol neurolysis can play a meaningful role in preserving joint movement in spasticity, neurotoxins have permitted a nuanced and focal approach to balancing muscle forces. It is possible to target a single finger flexor or an entire limb without the prospect of neuropathic pain as an unwanted outcome. Neurotoxins have also been shown to diminish the severity and frequency of migraine headaches, modulate bladder function in hyper-reflexic conditions, and assist in controlling the flow of saliva and sweat via glandular muscle relaxation. For so many, the use of these toxins has been life-changing, helping to restore movement and relieve pain.

It has long been a dream of Dr. Fatma Gul to leave a compendium of the knowledge she has gained over the past 30 years regarding the use of neurotoxins to manage spasticity and other disorders as the director of the Spasticity Management program at the University of Texas Southwestern Medical Center. She and her colleagues, Drs. Surendra Barshikar, Merrine Klakeel, and Amy Mathews, have labored over many weekends and nights, eating too much take-out and too many donuts, to produce this comprehensive yet pocket-sized treasure. This book will become an invaluable, dog-eared companion to many trainees and practitioners alike, traveling in white coat pockets and shoulder bags.

I'm very proud of our spasticity management team here at the University of Texas Southwestern and equally delighted that patients everywhere will benefit from their experience and wisdom.

Kathleen R. Bell, MD
Professor and Chair
Kimberly Clark Distinguished Chair in Mobility Research
University of Texas Southwestern Medical Center
Dallas, Texas

Preface

Practical Guide to Botulinum Toxin Injections is intended to be used as a quick and accessible reference for injectors during the course of their clinical practice. As practitioners of chemodenervation ourselves, we have been looking for an up-to-date, uniform resource in a convenient format, which is ultimately what led us to writing this pocketbook. The inclusion of visual and textual information for executing injection localization and suggested dosing for the four commercially available toxins makes this book a unique, one-stop resource. Our goal is that both novice and experienced injectors may use this pocketbook as a practical and evidence-based tool in the course of planning and executing injections.

As educators, this book will serve as a visual adjunct to bedside teaching. The authors of this book are all directly involved in educating medical trainees in the evaluation and management of spasticity. Despite a robust spasticity curriculum and hands-on experience, we still felt a need for a physical resource to help residents and fellows during the course of their training and as they started their careers. For novice injectors and medical trainees, performing botulinum toxin injections can seem daunting. Our hope is that, with the use of this book, knowledge can be consolidated into an accessible format, allowing providers to reinforce and sharpen previously learned skills.

Our senior author, Dr. Fatma Gul, started her private practice 35 years ago as a neuro-rehabilitation physiatrist. It did not take her long to realize that spasticity was often comorbid with many of the disorders she was treating. At that time, clinicians had limited resources for spasticity, which included rehabilitation modalities and anti-spasticity medications. As the field developed and new toxins became commercially available, Dr. Gul honed her expertise in the clinical application of this treatment. The junior faculty in our department have relied on the clinical experience and expertise of Dr. Gul to mentor the treatment of our most complicated patients. We wanted to create a uniform resource for current and future injectors that shared the benefits of this clinical experience as well as current, evidence-based medicine.

Writing a book is never an easy task, but the dedication, discipline, and hard work of this team of authors made it possible. Working as a team has been truly a wonderful, enjoyable, and fun experience for all of us. Seeing this project coming into fruition has been a dream come true. We dedicate this book to our families and all the current and future botulinum toxin injectors.

Surendra Barshikar, MD
Fatma Gul, MD, MSc
Merrine Klakeel, DO
Amy Mathews, MD

Abbreviation List

ABTA	abobotulinumtoxin A (Dysport®)
AD	autonomic dysreflexia
ADLs	activities of daily living
BoNT	botulinum neurotoxin
BPS	bladder pain syndrome
CD	cervical dystonia
CM	chronic migraine
CNS	central nervous system
DESD	detrusor external sphincter dyssynergia
DO	detrusor overactivity
DOI	detrusor overactivity incontinence
EMG	electromyography
e-stim	electrical stimulation
EUS	external urethral sphincter
FDA	U.S. Food and Drug Administration
HDSS	Hyperhidrosis Disease Severity Scale
HIT-6	Headache Impact Test 6
IBTA	incobotulinumtoxin A (Xeomin®)
IC	interstitial cystitis
IP	interphalangeal
LL	lower limb
MCP	metacarpophalangeal
MIDAS	Migraine Disability Assessment Scale
MPS	myofascial pain syndromes
MTP	myofascial trigger point
NS	normal saline
OBTA	onabotulinumtoxin A (Botox®)

pEMG	polymyographic electromyography
PREEMPT	Phase III Research Evaluating Migraine Prophylaxis Therapy
PROM	passive range of motion
RBTB	rimabotulinumtoxin B (Myobloc®/NeuroBloc®)
SCM	sternocleidomastoid
TOS	thoracic outlet syndrome
TWSTRS	Toronto Western Spasmodic Torticollis Rating Scale
UL	upper limb
UMNS	upper motor neuron syndrome
US	ultrasonography
WHO ICF	World Health Organization International Classification of Functioning, Disability and Health

Introduction

CHAPTER 1

Introduction to Botulinum Neurotoxin

Clostridium botulinum is a spore-forming gram-positive rod that is commonly found in soil and water. It produces a toxin called botulinum neurotoxin (BoNT) which is one of the most potent toxins known to mankind. Christian Andreas Justinus Kerner published the first case of botulism in 1817 and called it "sausage poison." He noted that it paralyzed the skeletal muscle function and the parasympathetic nervous system and proposed its use as a therapeutic agent in neurological diseases characterized by involuntary movements. The first clinical use was published in 1973 by Alan Scott in monkeys and later in 1977 in humans for treatment of strabismus.[1]

There are eight serotypes of BoNT: A, B, C, D, E, F, G, and H, out of which A and B have been used clinically (Table 1.1). Both BoNT A and B work by inhibiting release of acetylcholine from presynaptic terminals, but BoNT A acts on SNAP-25 while BoNT B

Table 1.1 Comparison of Botulinum Neurotoxins Used Clinically

Name	Onabotulinumtoxin A (OBTA)[1,3,4]	Abobotulinumtoxin A (ABTA)[1,5]	Incobotulinumtoxin A (IBTA)[1,6]	Rimabotulinumtoxin B (RBTB)[1,7]
Trade Name	Botox®	Dysport®	Xeomin®	Myobloc®/NeuroBloc®
Company	Allergan, USA	Ipsen, UK	Merz, Germany	Solstice Neurosciences, US WorldMeds, USA
Weight (kilodalton)	900 kD	500–900 kD	150 kD	700 kD
Shelf life	36 months	24 months	36 months	24 months
Storage temperature (Celsius)	Refrigerate 2°–8°	Refrigerate 2°–8°	Room temperature 20°–25°	Refrigerate 2°–8°
pH	7.4	7.4	7.4	5.6
Units/vial	50, 100, 200	300, 500	50, 100	2,500, 5,000, 10,000
Antigenic load ng/vial	0.8	Unknown	0.6	10.7

(continued)

Table 1.1 Comparison of Botulinum Neurotoxins Used Clinically (*continued*)

Name	Onabotulinumtoxin A (OBTA)[1,3,4]	Abobotulinumtoxin A (ABTA)[1,5]	Incobotulinumtoxin A (IBTA)[1,6]	Rimabotulinumtoxin B (RBTB)[1,7]
Immunogenicity rates[8]	0.2%–3.6%	0.9%–3.6%	0%–0.5%	18%–42.4%
FDA-approved indications	1. UL spasticity in adults 2. LL spasticity in adults 3. UL spasticity in pediatrics 4. LL spasticity in pediatrics 5. Cervical dystonia 6. Blepharospasm 7. Glabellar lines 8. Chronic migraine 9. Hyperhidrosis 10. Strabismus 11. Overactive bladder 12. Detrusor overactivity	1. UL spasticity in adults 2. LL spasticity in adults 3. LL spasticity in pediatrics 4. Cervical dystonia 5. Glabellar lines	1. UL spasticity in adults 2. Cervical dystonia 3. Blepharospasm 4. Glabellar lines 5. Chronic sialorrhea	1. Cervical dystonia 2. Chronic sialorrhea

FDA, U.S. Food and Drug Administration; LL, lower limb; UL, upper limb.

Source: Modified with permission from Jankovic J. Botulinum toxin: State of the art. *Mov Disord.* 2017;32(8):1131–1138. doi:10.1002/mds.27072

acts on synaptobrevin.[2] There are four commercially available toxins that are available for clinical use in the United States. FDA approval was first received in 1989 for the use of botulinum toxin A for the treatment of strabismus and blepharospasm.

Dilution and Reconstitution

All of the commercially available BoNT A toxins, OBTA, IBTA, and ABTA, come in a dried, powdered form that needs reconstitution with preservative-free 0.9% normal saline (NS) before injection. RBTB comes in sterile, colorless-to-light yellow solution that is ready to use.

OBTA and IBTA can be reconstituted using 1 to 4 mL of NS per vial depending on the indication and dilution needed. Generally higher dilution may be used for larger muscles in which diffusion is both tolerated and desirable. IBTA is usually reconstituted with 1.5 mL of NS for a 300-unit vial or with 2.5 mL of NS for a 500-unit vial; however, various dilution methods can be used depending on injector preference. Although RBTB comes ready to use, it may be further diluted if needed. Once reconstituted, ABTA should be used within 4 hours and OBTA and IBTA should be used within 24 hours. RBTB should be used within 4 hours of opening the product.

Dosing

Dosing of the toxins depends on clinical presentation, indication for use, and whether the patient is toxin naïve or not. Details of dosing are discussed in individual chapters for their respective indications. Although each of the botulinum toxins are different and their doses cannot be converted, approximate comparative dosing of different toxins have been mentioned in the literature to help guide injectors when switching toxins.[9]

> The muscle dosing amounts included in this book are suggestions but not absolute recommendations. The optimal starting dose, retreatment dose, and maximum dose should be based on clinical presentation and injector judgment.

Injection Technique and Guidance

Informed consent should be obtained by reviewing the risks and benefits of treatment with botulinum toxin with the patient before the procedure. A time out should be performed before the procedure commences. The procedure is performed under aseptic technique. Guidance for the procedure may be selected based on the user's skills, preferences, comfort level, and equipment available. Four common guidance techniques used are: anatomical localization, electromyography, electrical stimulation, and ultrasound. Many times, a combination of anatomical and other techniques is used. The benefits of anatomical technique are that it is rapid and does not need additional equipment. The other three techniques need specialized equipment but provide better accuracy. Ultrasound guidance requires additional equipment and needs an extra set of hands, but for skilled users this technique can provide better accuracy.[10] Studies have shown that in spite of clinical expertise there is only 30% to 70% localization accuracy using only anatomical guidance when confirmed by dissection or ultrasound.[10]

Contraindications for use of BoNT[3,5–7]:

- Hypersensitivity to any botulinum toxin preparation or to any of the components in the formulation
- Infection at the proposed site
- Urinary tract infections for bladder injections
- Neuromuscular disorders
- Pregnancy
- Concurrent use of aminoglycoside antibiotics

Adverse effects of use of BoNT[3,5–7]:

- Pain at injection site
- Flu-like syndrome
- Minor bleeding
- Respiratory muscle weakness and difficulty breathing
- Urinary tract infection, dysuria, urinary retention for bladder injections
- Dysphagia, upper respiratory infection, neck pain, dry mouth, headache when used for cervical dystonia
- Neck pain, eyebrow ptosis, and headache when used for migraine
- Upper respiratory tract infection, headache, eyelid edema, eyelid ptosis when used for glabellar lines

It is recommended to use clinical judgment when evaluating patients with neuromuscular disorders for BoNT injections. Based on animal studies, it is recommended that BoNT be avoided in pregnant women. We also recommend avoiding its use in breast-feeding women due to lack of sufficient studies available. Concurrent use of aminoglycoside antibiotics is known to potentiate the effects of botulinum toxin injections and should be avoided or extra care should be taken.

References

1. Jankovic J. Botulinum toxin: state of the art. *Mov Disord*. 2017;32(8): 1131–1138. doi:10.1002/mds.27072
2. Camargo CHF, Teive HAG. Use of botulinum toxin for movement disorders. *Drugs Context*. 2019;8:212586. doi:10.7573/dic.212586
3. Allergan. Botox [package insert]. Published July 2020. https://media .allergan.com/actavis/actavis/media/allergan-pdf-documents/product -prescribing/20190620-BOTOX-100-and-200-Units-v3-0USPI1145-v2 -0MG1145.pdf
4. Allergan. Botox [package insert] cosmetic. Published 2019. https://media .allergan.com/actavis/actavis/media/allergan-pdf-documents/product -prescribing/20190626-BOTOX-Cosmetic-Insert-72715US10-Med-Guide-v2 -0MG1145.pdf
5. Ipsen. Dysport [package insert]. Published September 2019. https://www.ipsen.com/websites/Ipsen_Online/wp-content/uploads/ sites/9/2020/01/09195739/S115_2019_09_25_sBLA_Approval_PMR_ Fulfilled_PI_MG_Sept-2019.pdf
6. Merz. Xeomin [package insert]. Published August 2020. https://dailymed .nlm.nih.gov/dailymed/fda/fdaDrugXsl.cfm?setid=ccdc3aae-6e2d-4cd0 -a51c-8375bfee9458&type=display
7. WorldMeds US. Myobloc [package insert]. Published August 2019. https:// myobloc.com/files/MYOBLOC_PI.pdf
8. Bellows S, Jankovic J. Immunogenicity associated with botulinum toxin treatment. *Toxins (Basel)*. 2019;11(9):491. doi:10.3390/toxins11090491
9. Safarpour Y, Jabbari B. Botulinum toxin treatment of movement disorders. *Curr Treat Options Neurol*. 2018;20(2):4. doi:10.1007/s11940-018-0488-3
10. Walker HW, Lee MY, Bahroo LB, Hedera P, Charles D. Botulinum toxin injection techniques for the management of adult spasticity. *PM R*. 2015;7(4):417–427. doi:10.1016/j.pmrj.2014.09.021

CHAPTER 2

Patient Evaluation

The upper motor neuron syndrome (UMNS) can be caused by a number of disease processes affecting the brain and/or spinal cord including stroke, traumatic brain injury, cerebral palsy, Parkinson's disease, multiple sclerosis, spinal cord injury, progressive neurologic diseases, and idiopathic causes. The UMNS is classically described as including negative and positive signs (Table 2.1). The interaction of these positive and negative symptoms, along with rheologic changes such as muscle or tendon shortening, lead to the individual clinical pattern observed in the patient.[1]

Table 2.1 Negative and Positive Features of the Upper Motor Neuron Syndrome

Negative Features	Positive Features
■ Weakness	■ Hyperreflexia
■ Loss of dexterity	■ Clonus
■ Impaired sensory perception	■ Positive Babinski sign
■ Fatigue	■ Spasms
	■ Mass synergy patterns
	■ Muscle overactivity/hypertonia (spasticity, dystonia, rigidity)

Source: Data from Lance JW. Symposium synopsis. In: Feldman RG, Young RR, Koella WP, eds. *Spasticity, Disordered Motor Control.* Symposia Specialists distributed by Year Book Medical Publishers; 1980:485–494; Lance JW. The control of muscle tone, reflexes, and movement: Robert Wartenberg Lecture. *Neurology.* 1980;30(12):1303–1313. doi:10.1212/WNL.30.12.1303; Mayer N. Spasticity and other signs of the upper motor neuron syndrome. In: Brashear A, Elovic E, eds. *Spasticity: Diagnosis and Management.* 2nd ed. Demos; 2016:17–32; Young RR. Spasticity: a review. *Neurology.* 1994;44(11 suppl 9):S12–S20. PubMed PMID: 7970006.

Classically, spasticity is defined as a "velocity-dependent increase in tonic stretch reflex (muscle tone) with exaggerated tendon jerks."[2] Dystonia is traditionally described as a sustained or intermittent muscle contraction, often causing involuntary postures or sustained movements with a twisting quality.[3] Rigidity is characterized as an increase in muscle tone to passive stretch throughout the muscle range of motion and is independent of velocity.[4]

Evaluation

Effective treatment of hypertonicity should be guided by patient interview and assessment of clinical and functional status, ideally in an interdisciplinary manner. The decision to treat hypertonicity is clinical and should be based on the potential to improve quality of life and minimize activity limitations or participation restrictions. Setting meaningful and realistic treatment goals is vital to the success of botulinum toxin interventions. It may be useful to discuss goals within the context of the World Health Organization's International Classification of Functioning, Disability and Health (Table 2.2). Practitioners may also consider using the Goal Attainment Scale in the assessment and follow-up of specific patient-centered goals.[5–8] Additionally, education should be provided so that UMNS impairments

Table 2.2 Goal Areas for Treatment of Spasticity Mapped onto WHO ICF

Symptom/Impairment	Goal Area
Pain or discomfort	■ Spasticity-related pain ■ Discomfort due to stiffness
Involuntary movement	■ Unwanted movements in reaction to use of other limbs ■ Spasms or dystonic movements
Contracture	■ Prevention of contracture and deformity ■ Tolerance of splinting and bracing
Activity/Function	**Goal Area**
Care of the affected limb	■ Maintaining hygiene and skin integrity ■ Dressing of the limb ■ Splint donning and doffing ■ Caregiver burden
Functional use of affected limb	■ Self-care ADLs ■ Instrumental ADLs ■ Vocational and avocational activities
Mobility	■ Transfers ■ Balance ■ Ambulation ■ Assistive device use for mobility
Other	**Goal Area**
Body image	■ Cosmesis and self-perception

ADLs, activities of daily living; WHO ICF, World Health Organization International Classification of Functioning, Disability and Health.

Source: Adapted from Sheean G, Lannin NA, Turner-Stokes L, Rawicki B, Snow BJ, Cerebral Palsy I. Botulinum toxin assessment, intervention and after-care for upper limb hypertonicity in adults: international consensus statement. *Eur J Neurol.* 2010;17(suppl 2):74–93. doi:10.1111/j.1468-1331 .2010.03129.x; Turner-Stokes L, Ashford S, Esquenazi A, et al. A comprehensive person-centered approach to adult spastic paresis: a consensus-based framework. *Eur J Phys Rehabil Med.* 2018;54(4):605–617. doi:10.23736/S1973-9087.17.04808-0

such as hypertonicity may respond to chemodenervation with botulinum toxin, while impairments such as weakness and sensory loss likely will not respond to these treatments.

In addition to goal-setting, the patient and caregiver interview may also include the following items which can impact treatment planning[9-11]:

- Etiology and chronicity of hypertonicity
- Assessment of previous treatments for spasticity and responses to these treatments
- Documentation of current therapies for hypertonia including stretching, splinting, serial casting, positioning, modalities, oral medications, phenol neurolysis, and/or intrathecal baclofen
- Assessment of contraindications and relative contraindications
- Identification of funding source

Examination should include[7,9]:

- Neurologic assessment noting positive and negative signs of UMNS with passive, active, and functional examinations
- Musculoskeletal examination including loss of range of motion and muscle bulk
- Evaluation for clinical factors that may confound or exacerbate hypertonicity such as pain, wounds, infections, and systemic stressors
- Identification of the location and distribution of hypertonicity—focal or generalized
- Notation of number of muscles involved

Scales

Scales may be used to facilitate communication among the treatment teams and for follow-up of treatment response.

Spasticity

The Modified Ashworth Scale is a six-point scale ranging from 0 to 4 (Table 2.3). It is used to describe muscle tone, specifically the resistance to passive muscle stretch felt by an examiner.[12,13]

Modified Tardieu Scale assesses hypertonicity with both slow and fast passive stretch, noting the quality and angle of muscle reaction (Table 2.4).[14,15]

Table 2.3 Modified Ashworth Scale

Grade	Description
0	No increase in muscle tone
1	Slight increase in muscle tone manifested by a catch and release at the end of the range of motion
1+	Slight increase in muscle tone manifested by a catch, followed by minimal resistance throughout the remainder (<50%) of the range of motion
2	More marked increase in muscle tone throughout >50% of the range of motion with joint being easily moved
3	Considerable increase in muscle tone, passive movement is difficult
4	Affected part is rigid in flexion or extension

Source: Reproduced with permission from Bohannon RW, Smith MB. Interrater reliability of a modified Ashworth scale of muscle spasticity. *Phys Ther.* 1987;67(2):206–207. doi:10.1093/ptj/67.2.206

Table 2.4 Modified Tardieu Scale

Angle of Muscle Reactions	
R1	Angle of muscle reaction/catch when stretching at fast velocity of V3
R2	Angle of muscle reaction/catch when stretching at slow velocity of V1
R2–R1	Spasticity angle: degrees of velocity-dependent hypertonicity
Speed Definitions: V1 = As slow as possible (slower than natural drop of limb falling under gravity) V2 = Speed of the limb segment falling under gravity V3 = As fast as possible (faster than natural drop of limb falling under gravity)	

Quality of Muscle Reaction	
Grade	Description
0	No resistance throughout the PROM
1	Slight resistance throughout the course of the PROM, no clear catch at precise angle
2	Distinctive catch at an angle with passive stretch, followed by release
3	Fatigable clonus (<10 seconds when maintaining pressure) occurring at a precise angle
4	Infatigable clonus (>10 seconds when maintain pressure) occurring at a precise angle

PROM, passive range of motion.
Source: Reproduced with permission from Boyd RN, Graham HK. Objective measurement of clinical findings in the use of botulinum toxin type A for the management of children with cerebral palsy. *Eur J Neurol.* 1999;6(S4):s23–s35. doi:10.1111/j.1468-1331.1999.tb00031.x

The Burke-Fahn-Marsden Dystonia Scale evaluates dystonia in nine body areas with scores ranging from 0 to 120 (Tables 2.5 and 2.6). For each body area, severity and provoking factor scores are given. The scores are multiplied together and with a weight to give a total score for each body region. Scores from each body region are summed to give the overall score.[16–18]

Table 2.5 Burke-Fahn-Marsden Dystonia Scale

Provoking Factors	
General	
0	No dystonia at rest or with action
1	Dystonia only with particular action
2	Dystonia with many actions
3	Dystonia on action of a distant part of body or intermittently at rest
4	Dystonia present at rest
Speech and swallowing	
1	Occasional, either or both
2	Frequent either
3	Frequent one and occasional other
4	Frequent both
Severity Factors	
Eyes	
0	No dystonia
1	Slight: Occasional blinking
2	Mild: Frequent blinking without prolonged spasms of eye closure
3	Moderate: Prolonged spasms of eyelid closure, but eyes open most of the time
4	Severe: Prolonged spasm of eyelid closure, with eyes closed at least 30% of the time
Mouth	
0	No dystonia present
1	Slight: Occasional grimacing or other mouth movements (e.g., jaw opened or clenched; tongue movement)
2	Mild: Movement present less than 50% of the time
3	Moderate: Dystonic movements or contractions present most of the time
4	Severe: Dystonic movements or contractions present most of the time
Speech and swallowing	
0	Normal
1	Slightly involved; speech easily understood or occasional choking
2	Some difficulty in understanding speech or frequent choking
3	Marked difficulty in understanding speech or inability to swallow firm foods
4	Complete or almost complete anarthria, or marked difficulty swallowing soft foods and liquids
Neck	
0	No dystonia present
1	Slight, occasional pulling
2	Obvious torticollis, but mild

(continued)

Table 2.5 Burke-Fahn-Marsden Dystonia Scale (*continued*)

3	Moderate pulling
4	Extreme pulling
Arm	
0	No dystonia present
1	Slight dystonia: Clinically insignificant
2	Mild: Obvious dystonia, but not disabling
3	Moderate: Able to grasp, with some manual function
4	Severe: No useful grasp
Trunk	
0	No dystonia present
1	Slight bending, clinically insignificant
2	Definite bending, but not interfering with standing or walking
3	Moderate bending, interfering with standing or walking
4	Extreme bending of trunk preventing standing or walking
Leg	
0	No dystonia present
1	Slight dystonia, but not causing impairment; clinically insignificant
2	Mild dystonia, walks briskly and unaided
3	Moderate dystonia, severely impairs walking or requires assistance
4	Severe dystonia, unable to stand or walk on involved leg

Source: Reproduced with permission from Burke RE, Fahn S, Marsden CD, Bressman SB, Moskowitz C, Friedman J. Validity and reliability of a rating scale for the primary torsion dystonias. *Neurology.* 1985;35(1):73–77. doi:10.1212/WNL.35.1.73

Table 2.6 Scoring for Burke-Fahn-Marsden Dystonia Scale

Region	Provoking Factor Score	Severity Factor Score	Weight	Weighted Score
Eyes	0–4	0–4	0.5	0–8
Mouth	0–4	0–4	0.5	0–8
Speech and swallowing	0–4	0–4	1.0	0–16
Neck	0–4	0–4	0.5	0–8
Right arm	0–4	0–4	1.0	0–16
Left arm	0–4	0–4	1.0	0–16
Trunk	0–4	0–4	1.0	0–16
Right leg	0–4	0–4	1.0	0–16
Left leg	0–4	0–4	1.0	0–16

Source: Modified from Comella CL, Leurgans S, Wuu J, Stebbins GT, Chmura T, Dystonia Study Global. Rating scales for dystonia: a multicenter assessment. *Mov Disord.* 2003;18(3):303–312. doi:10.1002/mds.10377

Other scales to consider for evaluation of dystonia are the Unified Dystonia Rating Scale and the Global Dystonia Rating Scale.[17]

Measures of voluntary activity and performance-based measures, such as the Box and Block Test or Fugl-Meyer, in addition to functional measures such as timed ambulation tests or functional independence measures, may also be considered in the assessment of hypertonicity. Assessment tools and scales for migraine, cervical dystonia, blepharospasm, and hyperhidrosis will be discussed elsewhere in this text.

References

1. Mayer N. Spasticity and other signs of the upper motor neuron syndrome. In: Brashear A, Elovic E, eds. *Spasticity: Diagnosis and Management*. 2nd ed. Demos; 2016:17–32.
2. Lance JW. Symposium synopsis. In: Feldman RG, Young RR, Koella WP, eds. *Spasticity, Disordered Motor Control*. Symposia Specialists distributed by Year Book Medical Publishers; 1980:485–494.
3. Fahn S. Concept and classification of dystonia. *Adv Neurol*. 1988;50:1–8. PubMed PMID: 3041755.
4. Gans B, Glenn MB. Introduction. In: Glenn MB, Whyte J, eds. *The Practical Management of Spasticity in Children and Adults*. Lea & Febiger; 1990:1–7.
5. Ashford S, Turner-Stokes L. Goal attainment for spasticity management using botulinum toxin. *Physiother Res Int*. 2006;11(1):24–34. doi:10.1002/pri.36
6. Turner-Stokes L, Ashford S, Esquenazi A, et al. A comprehensive person-centered approach to adult spastic paresis: a consensus-based framework. *Eur J Phys Rehabil Med*. 2018;54(4):605–617. doi:10.23736/S1973-9087.17.04808-0
7. Wissel J, Ward AB, Erztgaard P, et al. European consensus table on the use of botulinum toxin type A in adult spasticity. *J Rehabil Med*. 2009;41(1):13–25. doi:10.2340/16501977-0303
8. Sheean G, Lannin NA, Turner-Stokes L, Rawicki B, Snow BJ, Cerebral Palsy I. Botulinum toxin assessment, intervention and after-care for upper limb hypertonicity in adults: international consensus statement. *Eur J Neurol*. 2010;17 (suppl 2):74–93. doi:10.1111/j.1468-1331.2010.03129.x
9. Francisco GE. Botulinum toxin: dosing and dilution. *Am J Phys Med Rehabil*. 2004;83(10 suppl):S30–S37. doi:10.1097/01.PHM.0000141128.62598.81
10. Bell KR, Williams F. Use of botulinum toxin type A and type B for spasticity in upper and lower limbs. *Phys Med Rehabil Clin N Am*. 2003;14(4):821–835. doi:10.1016/S1047-9651(03)00064-0
11. Esquenazi A, Novak I, Sheean G, Singer BJ, Ward AB. International consensus statement for the use of botulinum toxin treatment in adults and children with neurological impairments—introduction. *Eur J Neurol*. 2010;17 (suppl 2):1–8. doi:10.1111/j.1468-1331.2010.03125.x
12. Ansari NN, Naghdi S, Arab TK, Jalaie S. The interrater and intrarater reliability of the Modified Ashworth Scale in the assessment of muscle spasticity: limb and muscle group effect. *NeuroRehabilitation*. 2008;23(3):231–237. doi:10.3233/NRE-2008-23304
13. Bohannon RW, Smith MB. Interrater reliability of a modified Ashworth scale of muscle spasticity. *Phys Ther*. 1987;67(2):206–207. doi:10.1093/ptj/67.2.206

14.   Ansari NN, Naghdi S, Hasson S, Azarsa MH, Azarnia S. The Modified Tardieu Scale for the measurement of elbow flexor spasticity in adult patients with hemiplegia. *Brain Inj*. 2008;22(13–14):1007–1012. doi:10.1080/02699050802530557

15.   Boyd RN, Graham HK. Objective measurement of clinical findings in the use of botulinum toxin type A for the management of children with cerebral palsy. *Eur J Neurol*. 1999;6(S4):s23–s35. doi:10.1111/j.1468-1331.1999.tb00031.x

16.   Comella CL, Leurgans S, Wuu J, Stebbins GT, Chmura T, Dystonia Study Global. Rating scales for dystonia: a multicenter assessment. *Mov Disord*. 2003;18(3):303–312. doi:10.1002/mds.10377

17.   Albanese A, Sorbo FD, Comella C, et al. Dystonia rating scales: critique and recommendations. *Mov Disord*. 2013;28(7):874–883. doi:10.1002/mds.25579

18.   Burke RE, Fahn S, Marsden CD, Bressman SB, Moskowitz C, Friedman J. Validity and reliability of a rating scale for the primary torsion dystonias. *Neurology*. 1985;35(1):73–77. doi:10.1212/WNL.35.1.73

PART II

Clinical Applications: Upper Limb Spasticity and Dystonia

CHAPTER 3

Muscles of the Pectoral Girdle and Shoulder

3.1 Pectoralis Minor

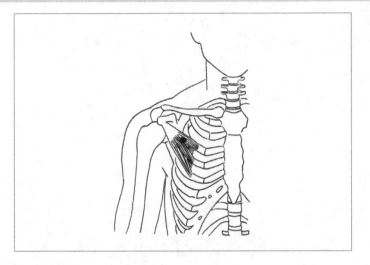

- *Muscle Origin:* Ribs 3–5
- *Muscle Insertion:* Coracoid process of the scapula
- *Muscle Action:* Depression of the shoulder, downward rotation of the scapula
- *Injection Localization:* In the midclavicular line anterior to the third rib. Needle will go through the pectoralis major.
- *Recommended Number of Injection Sites:* 1

	Botox® (units)	Dysport® (units)	Xeomin® (units)	Myobloc® (units)
Suggested Dose	10–40[1,2]	40–200[1]	10–40[1,2]	1,000–3,000*

*Author recommendation.

(continued)

INJECTION PEARLS AND PITFALLS

If the needle is inserted too superficially, then it will be in the pectoralis major. Minimize the risk of pneumothorax by palpating the rib prior to injection.

3.2 Pectoralis Major

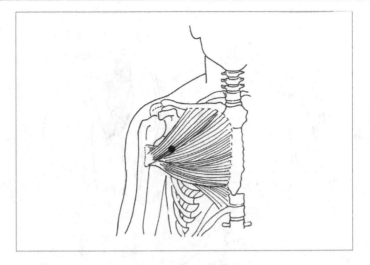

- *Muscle Origin:* Medial two-thirds of the clavicle, sternum, costal cartilages 1–6
- *Muscle Insertion:* Lateral lip of the intertubercular groove of the humerus
- *Muscle Action:* Adduction and medial rotation of the arm; clavicular fibers assist in flexion and sternocostal fibers assist in extension at the shoulder
- *Injection Localization:* Anterior axillary fold
- *Recommended Number of Injection Sites:* 1–3

	Botox (units)	Dysport (units)	Xeomin (units)	Myobloc (units)
Suggested Dose	20–150[1,3]	60–300[1,4]	20–100[1]	2,500–5,000[3]

INJECTION PEARLS AND PITFALLS

If the needle is inserted too deeply, then it will be in the coracobrachialis or pectoralis minor. If inserted too laterally, then it will be in the biceps brachii. There is a risk of pneumothorax if injected too deeply.

3.3 Deltoid

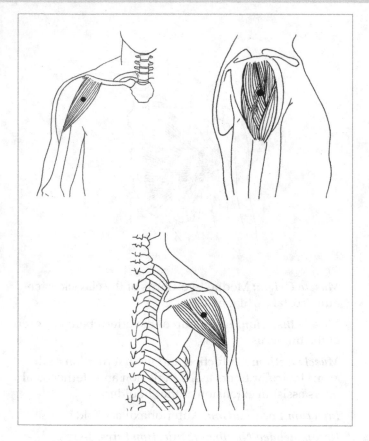

- *Muscle Origin:* Lateral third of the clavicle, acromion, spine of scapula
- *Muscle Insertion:* Deltoid tuberosity of the humerus
- *Muscle Action:* Anterior fibers assist with flexion and internal rotation, middle fibers assist with abduction, and posterior fibers assist with extension and external rotation of the shoulder
- *Injection Localization:*
  - Anterior fibers: 3 fingerbreadths below the anterior margin on the acromion

(continued)

- Middle fibers: Midway between the tip of the acromion and deltoid tubercle
- Posterior fibers: 2 fingerbreadths inferior to the posterior margin of the acromion
- *Recommended Number of Injection Sites:* 3

	Botox (units)	Dysport (units)	Xeomin (units)	Myobloc (units)
Suggested Dose	25–75[2]	20–300[1,2]	25–75[2]	1,000–3,000*

*Author recommendations.

INJECTION PEARLS AND PITFALLS

For the anterior deltoid, if the needle is inserted too medially or too deeply, then it will be in the coracobrachialis. For the posterior deltoid, if the needle is inserted too medially, then it will be in the teres minor. If inserted too deeply, then it will be in the long head of the triceps.

3.4 Supraspinatus

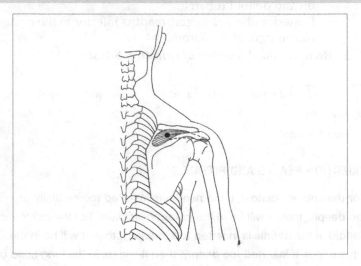

- **Muscle Origin:** Supraspinous fossa of the scapula
- **Muscle Insertion:** Greater tubercle of the humerus
- **Muscle Action:** Abduction of the shoulder
- **Injection Localization:** Supraspinous fossa superior to the middle of the spine of the scapula. Needle will pass through the trapezius muscle.
- **Recommended Number of Injection Sites:** 1

	Botox (units)	Dysport (units)	Xeomin (units)	Myobloc (units)
Suggested Dose	20–50[1,2]	60–200[2]	20–50[1,2]	1,000–2,500*

*Author recommendations.

INJECTION PEARLS AND PITFALLS

If the needle is inserted too superficially, then it will be in the trapezius.

3.5 Infraspinatus

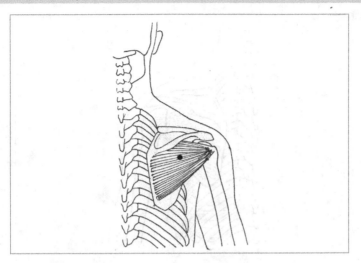

- *Muscle Origin:* Infraspinous fossa of the scapula
- *Muscle Insertion:* Greater tubercle of the humerus inferior to the supraspinatus insertion
- *Muscle Action:* External rotation of the shoulder
- *Injection Localization:* Infraspinous fossa 2 fingerbreadths below the midpoint of the spine of the scapula
- *Recommended Number of Injection Sites:* 1

	Botox (units)	Dysport (units)	Xeomin (units)	Myobloc (units)
Suggested Dose	20–60[1]	60–240[2]	20–60[1,2]	1,000–2,500*

*Author recommendations.

INJECTION PEARLS AND PITFALLS

If the needle is inserted too superficially, then it will be in the trapezius. If the needle is inserted too laterally, then it will be in the posterior deltoid.

3.6 Subscapularis

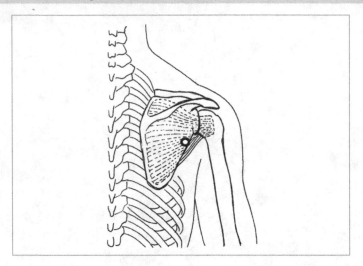

- *Muscle Origin:* Subscapular fossa of the scapula
- *Muscle Insertion:* Lesser tubercle and crest of the humerus
- *Muscle Action:* Internal rotation of the shoulder
- *Injection Localization:* Upper third of the lateral border of the scapula, anterior to the bone with the needle directed posteriorly. Please note: The illustration includes a dotted muscle and hollow circle as we want readers to understand that muscle is located anterior to the scapula.
- *Recommended Number of Injection Sites:* 1

	Botox (units)	Dysport (units)	Xeomin (units)	Myobloc (units)
Suggested Dose	25–100[3]	100–400[3]	15–100[2]	1,000–3,000[3]

INJECTION PEARLS AND PITFALLS

If the needle is inserted too anteriorly, then there is a high risk of pneumothorax. If the needle is inserted laterally, then it will be in the latissimus dorsi.

3.7 Teres Minor

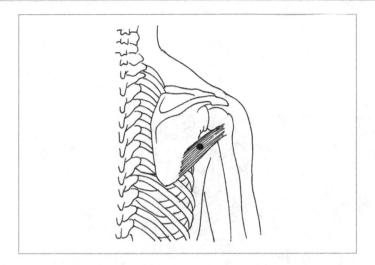

- *Muscle Origin:* Upper two-thirds of the lateral border of the scapula
- *Muscle Insertion:* Greater tubercle of the humerus inferior to the insertion of the infraspinatus
- *Muscle Action:* External rotation of the shoulder
- *Injection Localization:* One-third of the way between the acromion and the inferior angle of the scapula along the lateral border
- *Recommended Number of Injection Sites:* 1

	Botox (units)	Dysport (units)	Xeomin (units)	Myobloc (units)
Suggested Dose	20–50[1,2]	60–200[2]	20–50[1,2]	1,000–2,000*

*Author recommendations.

INJECTION PEARLS AND PITFALLS

If the needle is inserted too superficially, then it will be in the supraspinatus. If the needle is inserted too inferiorly, then it will be in the teres major. If the needle is inserted too superficially, then it will be in the trapezius. If the needle in inserted too medially, then it will be in the infraspinatus.

3.8 Teres Major

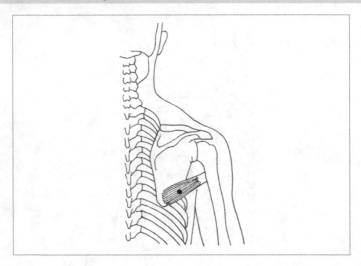

- *Muscle Origin:* Inferior angle of the scapula
- *Muscle Insertion:* Medial lip of the intertubercular groove of the humerus
- *Muscle Action:* Adduction, medial rotation, and extension of the shoulder
- *Injection Localization:* 3 fingerbreadths above the inferior angle of the scapula along the lateral border.
- *Recommended Number of Injection Sites:* 1

	Botox (units)	Dysport (units)	Xeomin (units)	Myobloc (units)
Suggested Dose	20–100[1,3]	60–200[2]	20–100[1,2]	1,000–3,000[3]

INJECTION PEARLS AND PITFALLS

If the needle is inserted too inferiorly, then it will be in the serratus anterior. If the needle is inserted too laterally, then it will be in the latissimus dorsi.

3.9 Serratus Anterior

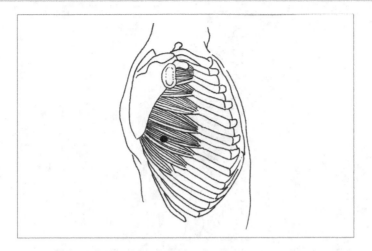

- *Muscle Origin:* Ribs 1–8
- *Muscle Insertion:* Medial border of the scapula and inferior angle
- *Muscle Action:* Protraction of the scapula, upward rotation of the glenoid cavity, holds the medial border of the scapula against the thoracic wall
- *Injection Localization:* One-half fingerbreadth lateral to the inferior angle of the scapula
- *Recommended Number of Injection Sites:* 1

	Botox (units)	Dysport (units)	Xcomin (units)	Myobloc (units)
Suggested Dose	25–70[1,2]	120–300[1]	25–70[1,2]	1,000–3,500*

*Author recommendations.

INJECTION PEARLS AND PITFALLS

If the needle is inserted too superficially, then it will be in the latissimus dorsi, and if inserted too cephalad it will be in the teres major. There is a risk of pneumothorax with deeper injection. Alternative injection technique involves multiple points along the origin at the ribs in divided doses.

3.10 Latissimus Dorsi

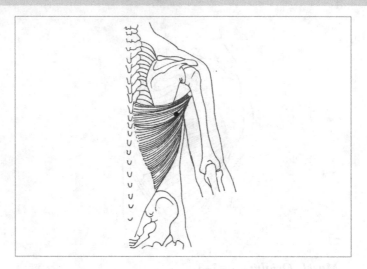

- *Muscle Origin:* Spinous process of the lower 6 thoracic, all lumbar and sacral vertebrae, posterior part of the iliac crest
- *Muscle Insertion:* Intertubercular groove of the humerus
- *Muscle Action:* Adduction, extension, and internal rotation of the shoulder
- *Injection Localization:* Along the posterior axillary fold, 3 fingerbreadths distal to the posterior axillary fold
- *Recommended Number of Injection Sites:* 1–3

	Botox (units)	Dysport (units)	Xeomin (units)	Myobloc (units)
Suggested Dose	25–150[3]	80–400[1,3]	25–150[2,3]	2,500–7,500[4]

INJECTION PEARLS AND PITFALLS

If the needle is inserted too medially, then it will be in the teres major.

3.11 Rhomboid Minor

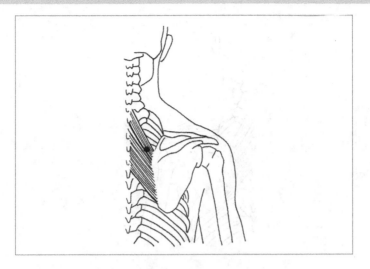

- *Muscle Origin:* Lower part of the ligamentum nuchae, spinous process of C7 and T1
- *Muscle Insertion:* Medial border of the scapula
- *Muscle Action:* Elevation and retraction of the scapula, downward rotation of the glenoid cavity
- *Injection Localization:* 1 fingerbreadth medial to the vertebral end of the scapular spine. Needle will pass through the upper trapezius.
- *Recommended Number of Injection Sites:* 1

	Botox (units)	Dysport (units)	Xeomin (units)	Myobloc (units)
Suggested Dose	20–50*	60–200*	20–50*	1,000–2,500*

*Author recommendations.

INJECTION PEARLS AND PITFALLS

If the needle is inserted too deeply, then it will be in the serratus posterior superior.

3.12 Rhomboid Major

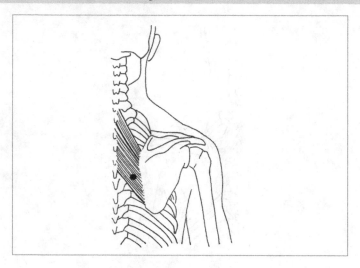

- *Muscle Origin:* Spinous process of T2–T5
- *Muscle Insertion:* Medial border of the scapula below the rhomboid minor
- *Muscle Action:* Elevation and retraction of the scapula, downward rotation of glenoid cavity
- *Injection Localization:* Inject 1 fingerbreadth medial to the medial border of the scapula at the midpoint between the scapular spine and inferior angle. Needle will pass through the middle trapezius.
- *Recommended Number of Injection Sites:* 1–2

	Botox (units)	Dysport (units)	Xeomin (units)	Myobloc (units)
Suggested Dose	20–60[1]	80–200[1,2]	20–60[1]	1,000–2,500*

*Author recommendations.

INJECTION PEARLS AND PITFALLS

If the needle is inserted too superficially, then it will be in the trapezius. If inserted too deeply, then it will be in the erector spinae muscles.

References

1. Jost W. *Pictorial Atlas of Botulinum Toxin Injection*. 2nd ed. Quintessence Publishing Co, Ltd; 2012.
2. Royal College of Physicians, British Society of Rehabilitation Medicine, Chartered Society of Physiotherapy, Association of Chartered Physiotherapists in Neurology and the Royal College of Occupational Therapists. Spasticity in adults: management using botulinum toxin. National guidelines. 2018. https://www.rcplondon.ac.uk/guidelines-policy/spasticity-adults-management-using-botulinum-toxin
3. Charles D, Gill CE. Neurotoxin injection for movement disorders. *Continuum (Minneap Minn)*. 2010;16(1 Movement Disorders):131–157. doi:10.1212/01.CON.0000348904.32834.70
4. Pathak MS, Nguyen HT, Graham HK, Moore AP. Management of spasticity in adults: practical application of botulinum toxin. *Eur J Neurol*. 2006;13 (suppl 1):42–50. doi:10.1111/j.1468-1331.2006.01444.x

CHAPTER 4

Muscles of the Upper Arm

4.1 Coracobrachialis

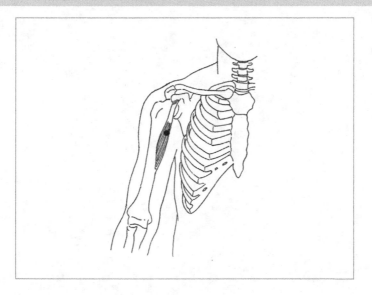

- *Muscle Origin:* Coracoid process of the scapula
- *Muscle Insertion:* Anteromedial surface of the humerus
- *Muscle Action:* Flexion at the shoulder and adduction of the arm
- *Injection Localization:* 4 fingerbreadths distal to the coracoid process along the volar aspect of the arm; insert needle to bone and withdraw
- *Recommended Number of Injection Sites:* 1

	Botox® (units)	Dysport® (units)	Xeomin® (units)	Myobloc® (units)
Suggested Dose	30–50[1]	120–200[1]	30–50[1]	1,000–2,500*

*Author recommendations.

(continued)

INJECTION PEARLS AND PITFALLS

If the needle is inserted too superiorly and medially, then it will be in the pectoralis complex. If the needle is inserted too superficially, then it will be in the biceps or anterior deltoid. If the needle is inserted too laterally, then it will be in the brachialis.

4.2 Biceps Brachii

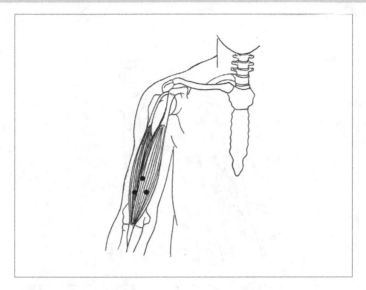

- *Muscle Origin:* Short head-tip of coracoid process of the scapula. Long head–supraglenoid tubercle of the scapula.

- *Muscle Insertion:* Radial tuberosity and bicipital aponeurosis

- *Muscle Action:* Flexion at the elbow, flexion at the shoulder, and supination of the forearm

- *Injection Localization:* Approach anteriorly at the junction of the middle and distal one-third of the upper arm in an inverted V pattern

- *Recommended Number of Injection Sites:* 2–4

	Botox (units)	Dysport (units)	Xeomin (units)	Myobloc (units)
Suggested Dose	25–200[2,3] (100–200)[†,4]	60–400[5,6] (200–400)[†,7]	20–200[5] (50–200)[†,8]	1,500–5,000[2]

†Denotes FDA-approved indication.

INJECTION PEARLS AND PITFALLS

If the needle is inserted too deeply, then it will be in the brachialis.

4.3 Brachialis

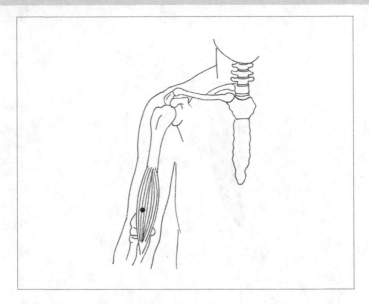

- *Muscle Origin:* Lower half of the anterior surface of the humerus, intermuscular septa
- *Muscle Insertion:* Ulnar tuberosity
- *Muscle Action:* Flexion at the elbow
- *Injection Localization:* 2 fingerbreadths proximal to the elbow crease lateral to the tendon and bulk of the biceps.
- *Recommended Number of Injection Sites:* 1–4

	Botox (units)	Dysport (units)	Xeomin (units)	Myobloc (units)
Suggested Dose	20–100[5,6]	50–400[1,5]	20–75[1,5]	1,500–5,000[2]
		(200–400)[†,7]	(25–100)[†,8]	

†Denotes FDA-approved indication.

INJECTION PEARLS AND PITFALLS

If the needle is inserted too medially, then it will be in the biceps.

4.4 Triceps Brachii

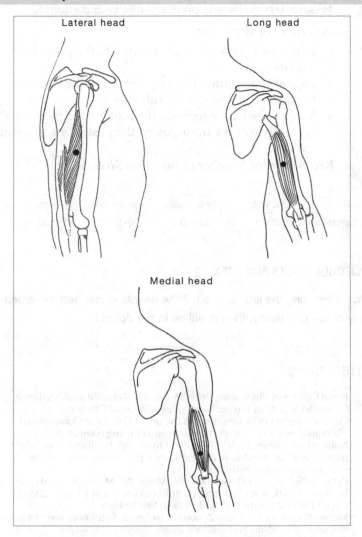

Lateral head

Long head

Medial head

- *Muscle Origin:* Long head—infraglenoid tubercle of the scapula. Lateral head—posterior surface of the humerus and lateral to the groove of the radial nerve and intermuscular septum. Medial head—posterior surface of the humerus below and medial to the groove of the radial nerve and intermuscular septa

(continued)

- *Muscle Insertion:* Proximal end of the olecranon
- *Muscle Action:* Extension at the elbow and shoulder
- *Injection Localization:*
  - Long head: 4 fingerbreadths distal to the posterior axillary fold
  - Lateral head: Immediately posterior to the insertion of the deltoid on the deltoid tubercle
  - Medial head: 3 fingerbreadths proximal to the medial epicondyle of the humerus on the posterior surface of the arm
- *Recommended Number of Injection Sites:* 1–3

	Botox (units)	Dysport (units)	Xeomin (units)	Myobloc (units)
Suggested Dose	30–200[5,6]	100–400[1,6]	30–100[1,5]	2,500–5,000[6]

INJECTION PEARLS AND PITFALLS

When injecting the lateral head, if the needle is inserted too anteriorly or too proximally, then it will be in the deltoid.

References

1. Royal College of Physicians, British Society of Rehabilitation Medicine, Chartered Society of Physiotherapy, Association of Chartered Physiotherapists in Neurology and the Royal College of Occupational Therapists. Spasticity in adults: management using botulinum toxin. National guidelines. Royal College of Physicians. Published March 2018. https://www.rcplondon.ac.uk/guidelines-policy/spasticity-adults-management-using-botulinum-toxin
2. Pathak MS, Nguyen HT, Graham HK, Moore AP. Management of spasticity in adults: practical application of botulinum toxin. *Eur J Neurol.* 2006;13 (suppl 1):42–50. doi:10.1111/j.1468-1331.2006.01444.x
3. Moeini-Naghani I, Hashemi-Zonouz T, Jabbari B. Botulinum toxin treatment of spasticity in adults and children. *Semin Neurol.* 2016;36(1):64–72. doi:10.1055/s-0036-1571847
4. Allergan. Botox [package insert]. Published July 2020. https://media.allergan.com/actavis/actavis/media/allergan-pdf-documents/product-prescribing/20190620-BOTOX-100-and-200-Units-v3-0USPI1145-v2-0MG1145.pdf
5. Jost W. *Pictorial Atlas of Botulinum Toxin Injection.* 2nd ed. Quintessence Publishing Co, Ltd; 2012.

6. Charles D, Gill CE. Neurotoxin injection for movement disorders. *Continuum (Minneap Minn)*. 2010;16(1 Movement Disorders):131–157. doi:10.1212/01.CON.0000348904.32834.70
7. Ipsen. Dysport [package insert]. Published September 2019. https://www.ipsen.com/websites/Ipsen_Online/wp-content/uploads/sites/9/2020/01/09195739/S115_2019_09_25_sBLA_Approval_PMR_Fulfilled_PI_MG_Sept-2019.pdf
8. Merz. Xeomin [package insert]. Published August 2020. https://dailymed.nlm.nih.gov/dailymed/fda/fdaDrugXsl.cfm?setid=ccdc3aae-6e2d-4cd0-a51c-8375bfee9458&type=display

CHAPTER 5

Muscles of the Forearm

5.1 Brachioradialis

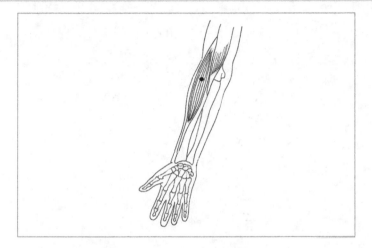

- *Muscle Origin:* Lateral supracondylar ridge of the humerus, lateral intermuscular septum of the arm
- *Muscle Insertion:* Lateral side of the distal end of the radius
- *Muscle Action:* Flexion at the elbow
- *Injection Localization:* 1 to 2 fingerbreadths distal to the elbow crease midway between the biceps tendon and lateral epicondyle
- *Recommended Number of Injection Sites:* 1–3

	Botox® (units)	Dysport® (units)	Xeomin® (units)	Myobloc® (units)
Suggested Dose	25–100[1]	75–300[1] (100–200)[†,2]	20–60[3,4] (25–100)[†,5]	1,000–3,750[1,6]

†Denotes FDA-approved indication.

(continued)

INJECTION PEARLS AND PITFALLS

If the needle is inserted too laterally, then it will be in the extensor carpi radialis longus.

5.2 Supinator

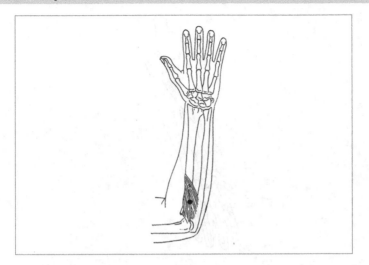

- *Muscle Origin:* Posterolateral surface of the ulna below the radial notch, lateral epicondyle, and radial and ulnar collateral ligaments
- *Muscle Insertion:* Lateral and adjacent posterior and anterior aspect of the proximal shaft of the radius
- *Muscle Action:* Supination of the forearm
- *Injection Localization:* Radial to the most distal part of the insertion of the biceps tendon. The needle will pass through the extensor digitorum communis.
- *Recommended Number of Injection Sites:* 1

	Botox (units)	Dysport (units)	Xeomin (units)	Myobloc (units)
Suggested Dose	20–50*	50–160[3]	20–50*	1,000–2,500*

*Author recommendations.

INJECTION PEARLS AND PITFALLS

If the needle is inserted too medially, then it will be in the brachioradialis.

5.3 Pronator Teres

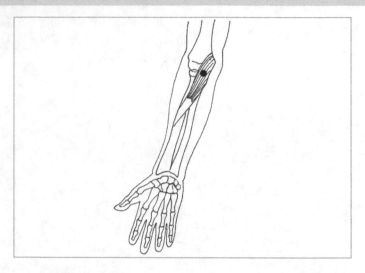

- *Muscle Origin:* Medial epicondyle of the humerus, coronoid process of the ulna
- *Muscle Insertion:* Lateral surface of the midshaft of the radius
- *Muscle Action:* Pronation of the forearm
- *Injection Localization:* 2 fingerbreadths distal to the midpoint of the line connecting the biceps tendon and medial epicondyle
- *Recommended Number of Injection Sites:* 1–2

	Botox (units)	Dysport (units)	Xeomin (units)	Myobloc (units)
Suggested Dose	25–75[1]	100–200[†,2]	25–75[†,5]	1,000–2,500[1]

[†]Denotes FDA-approved indication.

INJECTION PEARLS AND PITFALLS

If the needle is inserted too medially, then it will be in the flexor carpi radialis.

5.4 Pronator Quadratus

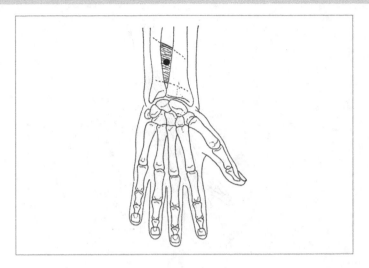

- *Muscle Origin:* Distal fourth of the anterior surface of the ulna
- *Muscle Insertion:* Distal part of the anterior surface of the radius
- *Muscle Action:* Pronation of the forearm
- *Injection Localization:* 3 fingerbreadths proximal to the midpoint of the line connecting the radial and ulnar styloid dorsally. Needle will pass through the interosseous membrane.
- *Recommended Number of Injection Sites:* 1

	Botox (units)	Dysport (units)	Xeomin (units)	Myobloc (units)
Suggested Dose	10–50[1]	30–120[3]	10–30[3]	1,000–2,500[1]

INJECTION PEARLS AND PITFALLS

If the needle is inserted too deeply, then it will be in the flexor digitorum superficialis.

5.5 Flexor Carpi Radialis

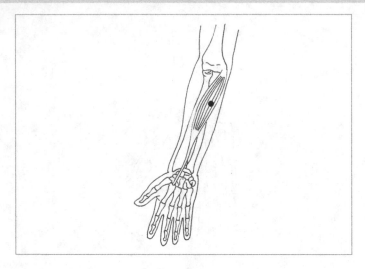

- *Muscle Origin:* Medial epicondyle of the humerus
- *Muscle Insertion:* Volar surface of the base of the second metacarpal
- *Muscle Action:* Flexion and radial deviation at the wrist
- *Injection Localization:* 3 to 4 fingerbreadths below the midpoint of the line connecting the medial epicondyle and the biceps tendon
- *Recommended Number of Injection Sites:* 1

	Botox (units)	Dysport (units)	Xeomin (units)	Myobloc (units)
Suggested Dose	15–100[1]	50–225[1]	25–100[†,5]	1,000–3,000[1]
	(12.5–50)[†,7]	(100–200)[†,2]		

[†]Denotes FDA-approved dosing.

INJECTION PEARLS AND PITFALLS

If the needle is inserted too deeply, then it will be in the flexor digitorum superficialis or flexor pollicis longus. If the needle is inserted too laterally, then it will be in the pronator teres. If the needle is inserted too medially, then it will be in the palmaris longus.

5.6 Flexor Carpi Ulnaris

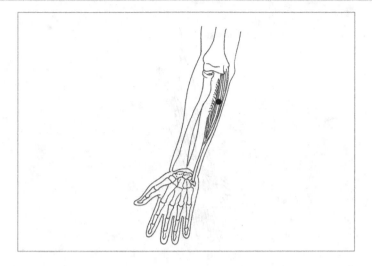

- *Muscle Origin:* Medial epicondyle of the humerus, proximal two-thirds of the posterior surface of the ulna
- *Muscle Insertion:* Pisiform bone
- *Muscle Action:* Flexion and ulnar deviation at the wrist
- *Injection Localization:* 2 fingerbreadths volar to the ulna at the junction of the proximal and middle thirds of the forearm
- *Recommended Number of Injection Sites:* 1–2

	Botox (units)	Dysport (units)	Xeomin (units)	Myobloc (units)
Suggested Dose	20–75[6]	60–225[1]	20–70[4]	1,000–3,000[1]
	(12.5–50)[†,7]	(100–200)[†,2]	(20–100)[†,5]	

[†]Denotes FDA-approved indication.

INJECTION PEARLS AND PITFALLS

If the needle is inserted too deeply, it will be in the flexor digitorum profundus.

5.7 Palmaris Longus

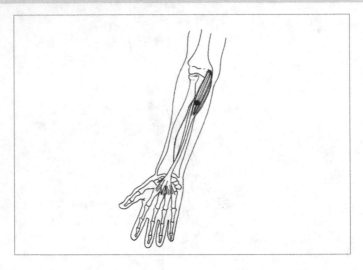

- *Muscle Origin:* Medial epicondyle of the humerus
- *Muscle Insertion:* Palmar aponeurosis
- *Muscle Action:* Flexion at the wrist
- *Injection Localization:* Draw a line joining the medial epicondyle and middle of the volar surface of the wrist. Inject at the junction of the upper and the middle thirds along this line.
- *Recommended Number of Injection Sites:* 1

	Botox (units)	Dysport (units)	Xeomin (units)	Myobloc (units)
Suggested Dose	10–25*	30–75*	10–25*	500–1,500*

*Author recommendations.

INJECTION PEARLS AND PITFALLS

If the needle is inserted too medially, it will be in the flexor car-pi ulnaris. If it is inserted too laterally it will be in the flexor carpi radialis. If it is inserted too deeply it will be in the flexor digitorum superficialis.

5.8 Extensor Carpi Radialis Longus and Brevis

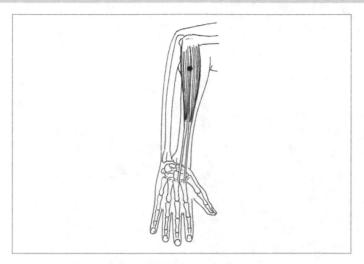

- *Muscle Origin:* Longus—lateral supracondylar ridge and lateral intermuscular septa, lateral epicondyle of the humerus. Brevis—lateral epicondyle of the humerus, intermuscular septa

- *Muscle Insertion:* Longus—dorsal surface of the base of the second metacarpal. Brevis—dorsal surface of the base of the third metacarpal

- *Muscle Action:* Extension and radial deviation at the wrist

- *Injection Localization:* 2 fingerbreadths distal to the lateral epicondyle

- *Recommended Number of Injection Sites:* 1

	Botox (units)	Dysport (units)	Xeomin (units)	Myobloc (units)
Suggested Dose	20–40[3]	60–160[3]	20–40[3]	1,000–2,500[6]

INJECTION PEARLS AND PITFALLS

If the needle is injected too deeply, then it will be in the supinator. Extensor carpi radialis longus and brevis have been mentioned together as it is difficult to separate them using EMG guidance.

5.9 Extensor Carpi Ulnaris

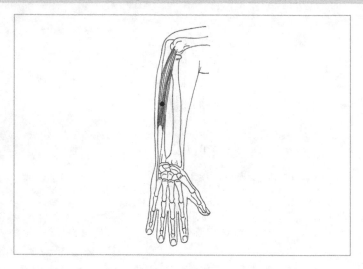

- *Muscle Origin:* Lateral epicondyle of the humerus, proximal half of the posterior border of the ulna
- *Muscle Insertion:* Dorsal surface of the base of the fifth metacarpal
- *Muscle Action:* Extension and ulnar deviation at the wrist
- *Injection Localization:* In the middle of the forearm just above the shaft of the ulna
- *Recommended Number of Injection Sites:* 1

	Botox (units)	Dysport (units)	Xeomin (units)	Myobloc (units)
Suggested Dose	20–40[3]	60–160[3]	20–40[3]	1,000–2,500*

*Author recommendations.

INJECTION PEARLS AND PITFALLS

If the needle is inserted too radially, then it will be in the extensor carpi radialis longus.

5.10 Flexor Digitorum Superficialis

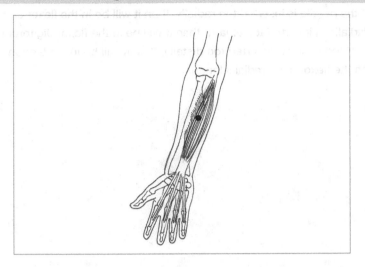

- *Muscle Origin:* Medial epicondyle of the humerus, medial aspect of the coronoid process of the ulna, proximal half of the radius distal to the radial tuberosity
- *Muscle Insertion:* Base of the middle phalanx of the medial 4 digits
- *Muscle Action:* Flexion at the proximal interphalangeal joint; assists with flexion at the metacarpophalangeal joint for digits 2 to 5 and the wrist
- *Injection Localization:* Grasp with injectors, palm to volar surface of the subject's wrist. Point the index finger toward the biceps tendon and insert the needle just ulnarly to the tip of the index finger. The needle will travel through the palmaris longus.
- *Recommended Number of Injection Sites:* 1–2

	Botox (units)	Dysport (units)	Xeomin (units)	Myobloc (units)
Suggested Dose	20–75[1]	50–225[1]	20–60[4]	1,000–3,000[1]
	(30–50)[†,7]	(100–200)[†,2]	(20–100)[†,5]	

[†]Denotes FDA-approved dosing.

(continued)

INJECTION PEARLS AND PITFALLS

If the needle is inserted too radially, then it will be in the flexor carpi radialis. If inserted too ulnarly, then it will be in the flexor digitorum profundus. If it is inserted too distally, then it will be in the tendon on the flexor carpi radialis longus.

5.11 Flexor Digitorum Profundus

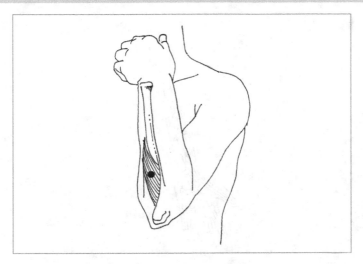

- *Muscle Origin:* Anterior and medial surfaces of the proximal two-thirds of the ulna, interosseous membrane, and aponeurosis of the flexor carpi ulnaris
- *Muscle Insertion:* Distal phalanx of the medial 4 digits
- *Muscle Action:* Flexion at the dorsal interphalangeal joint; assists with flexion at the proximal interphalangeal and metacarpophalangeal joint of digits 2 to 5 and the wrist.
- *Injection Localization:* 4 fingerbreadths distal to the olecranon off the shaft of the ulna
- *Recommended Number of Injection Sites:* 1–2

	Botox (units)	Dysport (units)	Xeomin (units)	Myobloc (units)
Suggested Dose	20–75[1]	50–225[1]	20–60[4]	1,000–3,000[1]
	(30–50)[†,7]	(100–200)[†,2]	(25–100)[†,5]	

[†]Denotes FDA-approved dosing.

INJECTION PEARLS AND PITFALLS

If the needle is inserted too volarly, then it will be in the flexor carpi ulnaris.

5.12 Flexor Pollicis Longus

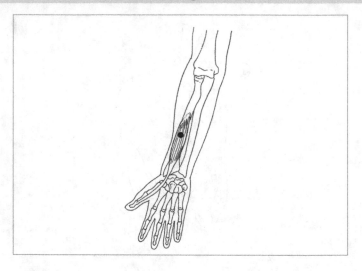

- **Muscle Origin:** Anterior surface of the middle half of the radius and interosseous membrane
- **Muscle Insertion:** Distal phalanx of the thumb
- **Muscle Action:** Flexion of the thumb at the interphalangeal joint
- **Injection Localization:** In the middle of the forearm just volar to the radius. The needle will pass through the flexor carpi radialis and flexor digitorum superficialis.
- **Recommended Number of Injection Sites:** 1

	Botox (units)	Dysport (units)	Xeomin (units)	Myobloc (units)
Suggested Dose	10–30[1] (20)[†,7]	30–120[3]	10–30[3] (10–50)[†,5]	1,000–2,500[1]

[†]Denotes FDA-approved indication.

INJECTION PEARLS AND PITFALLS

If the needle in inserted too superficially, then it will be in the flexor digitorum superficialis.

5.13 Extensor Digitorum Communis

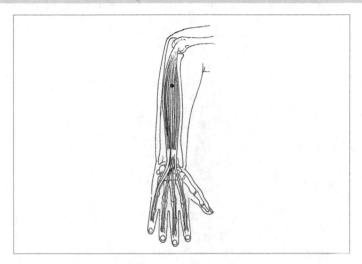

- *Muscle Origin:* Lateral epicondyle of the humerus
- *Muscle Insertion:* Dorsal surface of the middle and distal phalanges of the medial 4 digits
- *Muscle Action:* Extension of digits 2 to 5
- *Injection Localization:* On the dorsal aspect of the forearm at the junction of the proximal and middle thirds midway between the radius and ulna
- *Recommended Number of Injection Sites:* 1–2

	Botox (units)	Dysport (units)	Xeomin (units)	Myobloc (units)
Suggested Dose	20–40[3,4]	60–160[3]	20–40[3,4]	1,000–2,500*

*Author recommendations.

INJECTION PEARLS AND PITFALLS

If the needle is inserted too deeply, then it will be in the extensor pollicis longus. If the needle is inserted too medially, then it will be in the extensor carpi radialis brevis. If it is inserted too laterally, it will be in the extensor carpi ulnaris.

5.14 Extensor Indicis

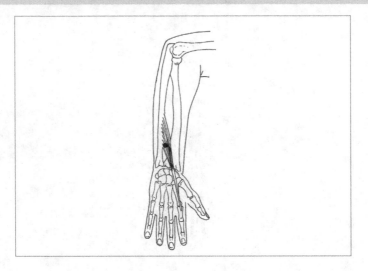

- *Muscle Origin:* Posterior surface of the ulna, interosseous membrane
- *Muscle Insertion:* Extensor expansion of the index finger
- *Muscle Action:* Extension and adduction of the index finger
- *Injection Localization:* 2 fingerbreadths proximal to the ulnar styloid just radial to the ulna on the dorsal aspect
- *Recommended Number of Injection Sites:* 1

	Botox (units)	Dysport (units)	Xeomin (units)	Myobloc (units)
Suggested Dose	10–30[3,4]	30–120[3,4]	10–30[3,4]	500–1,500*

*Author recommendations.

INJECTION PEARLS AND PITFALLS

If the needle is inserted too radially, then it will be in the abductor pollicis longus. If the needle is inserted too proximally, then it will be in the extensor digitorum communis.

5.15 Extensor Pollicis Brevis

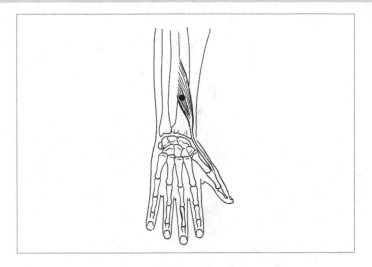

- *Muscle Origin:* Posterior surface of the radius
- *Muscle Insertion:* Dorsal aspect of the proximal phalanx of the thumb
- *Muscle Action:* Extension of the thumb at the metacarpophalangeal joint
- *Injection Localization:* Four fingerbreadths proximal to the wrist along the ulnar side of the radius on the dorsal side of the forearm
- *Recommended Number of Injection Sites:* 1

	Botox (units)	Dysport (units)	Xeomin (units)	Myobloc (units)
Suggested Dose	5–25[3,4,8]	20–80[3,4,8]	5–25[3,4]	500–1,000*

*Author recommendations.

INJECTION PEARLS AND PITFALLS

If the needle is inserted too superficially, then it will be in the extensor digitorum communis. If the needle is inserted too proximally, then it will be in the abductor pollicis longus.

5.16 Extensor Pollicis Longus

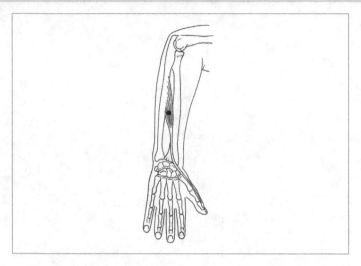

- *Muscle Origin:* Posterior surface of the middle-third of the ulna
- *Muscle Insertion:* Dorsal aspect of the distal phalanx of the thumb
- *Muscle Action:* Extension of the thumb at the metacarpophalangeal and interphalangeal joints
- *Injection Localization:* Dorsal side of the forearm, midway between the elbow and wrist, along the radial side of the ulna
- *Recommended Number of Injection Sites:* 1

	Botox (units)	Dysport (units)	Xeomin (units)	Myobloc (units)
Suggested Dose	10–30[3,4,8]	20–100[3,4,8]	10–20[3,4]	1,000–2,000*

*Author recommendations.

INJECTION PEARLS AND PITFALLS

If the needle is inserted too superficially, then it will be in the extensor carpi ulnaris. If the needle is inserted too ulnar, then it will be in the extensor digitorum communis.

5.17 Abductor Pollicis Longus

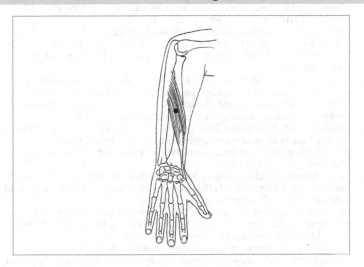

- *Muscle Origin:* Posterior surface of the ulna, radius, and interosseous membrane
- *Muscle Insertion:* Base of the first metacarpal
- *Muscle Action:* Abduction at the carpometacarpal joint and extension of the thumb
- *Injection Localization:* Dorsal side of the forearm, midway between the elbow and wrist, over the shaft of the radius
- *Recommended Number of Injection Sites:* 1–2

	Botox (units)	Dysport (units)	Xeomin (units)	Myobloc (units)
Suggested Dose	5–20[4,9]	20–80[4]	5–20[4]	500–1,000[6]

INJECTION PEARLS AND PITFALLS

If the needle is inserted too superficially, then it will be in the extensor digitorum communis. If the needle is inserted too proximally, then it will be in the extensor carpi radialis brevis. If the needle is inserted too distally, then it will be in the extensor pollicis brevis.

References

1. Charles D, Gill CE. Neurotoxin injection for movement disorders. *Continuum (Minneap Minn)*. 2010;16(1 Movement Disorders):131–157. doi:10.1212/01.CON.0000348904.32834.70

2. Ipsen. Dysport [package insert]. Published September 2019. https://www.ipsen.com/websites/Ipsen_Online/wp-content/uploads/sites/9/2020/01/09195739/S115_2019_09_25_sBLA_Approval_PMR_Fulfilled_PI_MG_Sept-2019.pdf

3. Royal College of Physicians, British Society of Rehabilitation Medicine, Chartered Society of Physiotherapy, Association of Chartered Physiotherapists in Neurology and the Royal College of Occupational Therapists. Spasticity in adults: management using botulinum toxin. National guidelines. RCP. Published 2018. https://www.rcplondon.ac.uk/guidelines-policy/spasticity-adults-management-using-botulinum-toxin

4. Jost W. *Pictorial Atlas of Botulinum Toxin Injection*. 2nd ed. Quintessence Publishing Co, Ltd; 2012.

5. Merz. Xeomin [package insert]. Published August 2020. https://dailymed.nlm.nih.gov/dailymed/fda/fdaDrugXsl.cfm?setid=ccdc3aae-6e2d-4cd0-a51c-8375bfee9458&type=display

6. Pathak MS, Nguyen HT, Graham HK, Moore AP. Management of spasticity in adults: practical application of botulinum toxin. *Eur J Neurol*. 2006;13 (suppl 1):42–50. doi:10.1111/j.1468-1331.2006.01444.x

7. Allergan. Botox [package insert]. Published July 2020. https://media.allergan.com/actavis/actavis/media/allergan-pdf-documents/product-prescribing/20190620-BOTOX-100-and-200-Units-v3-0USPI1145-v2-0MG1145.pdf

8. Sheean G, Lannin NA, Turner-Stokes L, et al. Botulinum toxin assessment, intervention and after-care for upper limb hypertonicity in adults: international consensus statement. *Eur J Neurol*. 2010;17 (suppl 2):74–93. doi:10.1111/j.1468-1331.2010.03129.x

9. Simpson DM, Patel AT, Alfaro A, et al. OnabotulinumtoxinA injection for poststroke upper-limb spasticity: guidance for early injectors from a Delphi panel process. *PM R*. 2017;9(2):136–148. doi:10.1016/j.pmrj.2016.06.016

CHAPTER 6

Muscles of the Hand

6.1 Flexor Pollicis Brevis

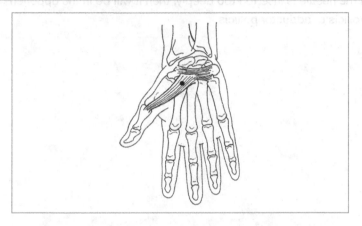

- *Muscle Origin:* Superficial head-flexor retinaculum and trapezium. Deep head—trapezoid and capitate
- *Muscle Insertion:* Superficial and deep heads—base of the proximal phalanx of the thumb
- *Muscle Action:* Flexion of the thumb at the carpometacarpal and metacarpophalangeal (MCP) joint
- *Injection Localization:*
  - Superficial Head: Along a line drawn from the first MCP joint and pisiform, the needle is inserted at the junction between the middle and radial third of the line to a depth of 1/2".
  - Deep Head: Same point as the superficial head, but 3/4" deep

(continued)

■ *Recommended Number of Injection Sites:* 1

	Botox® (units)	Dysport® (units)	Xeomin® (units)	Myobloc® (units)
Suggested Dose	5–25[1,2]	20–50[†,3]	10–30[†,4]	250–1,500[5]

[†]Denotes FDA-approved dosing.

INJECTION PEARLS AND PITFALLS

If the needle is inserted too deeply, then it will be in the opponens pollicis or adductor pollicis.

6.2 Adductor Pollicis

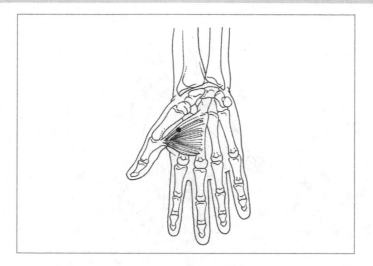

- *Muscle Origin:* Transverse head—third metacarpal; oblique head—capitate, trapezoid, trapezium, bases of second to third metacarpals
- *Muscle Insertion:* Base of proximal phalanx of the thumb
- *Muscle Action:* Adduction of the thumb
- *Injection Localization:* Proximal end of the first metacarpal in the first web space
- *Recommended Number of Injection Sites:* 1

	Botox (units)	Dysport (units)	Xeomin (units)	Myobloc (units)
Suggested Dose	2.5–40[2,5–9] (20)[†,10]	25–100[2,5,8,9]	2.5–40[8,9,11] (5–30)[†,4]	250–1,500[5,12]

[†]Denotes FDA-approved dosing.

INJECTION PEARLS AND PITFALLS

If the needle is inserted too dorsal, it will be in the first dorsal interosseous. If the needle is inserted too volar, it will be in the opponens pollicis.

6.3 Opponens Pollicis

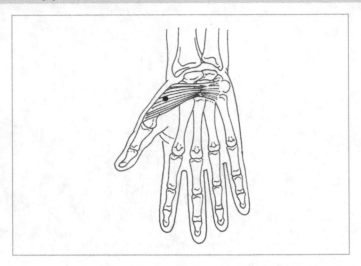

- ■ *Muscle Origin:* Flexor retinaculum, trapezium
- ■ *Muscle Insertion:* First metacarpal
- ■ *Muscle Action:* Opposition of the thumb
- ■ *Injection Localization:* Midpoint of a line drawn between the radial aspect of the carpometacarpal and first MCP joints, depth of 1/2″ to 3/4″
- ■ *Recommended Number of Injection Sites:* 1

	Botox (units)	Dysport (units)	Xeomin (units)	Myobloc (units)
Suggested Dose	2.5–25[6,8]	10–40[8]	2.5–25[8,11]	500–1,500[12]

INJECTION PEARLS AND PITFALLS

If the needle is inserted too deeply, then it will be in the adductor pollicis. If the needle is inserted too medially, then it will be in the abductor pollicis brevis.

6.4 Dorsal Interossei

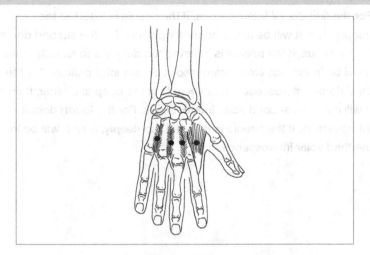

- *Muscle Origin:* Two adjacent metacarpals
- *Muscle Insertion:* #1, #2—radial side of the proximal phalanx of the index and middle finger, respectively. #3, #4—ulnar side of the proximal phalanx of the middle and ring finger, respectively
- *Muscle Action:* Abduction of digits 2, 3, 4, flexion at the MCP joints; extension of the interphalangeal (IP) joints
- *Injection Localization:* Draw a line perpendicular to the long axis of the hand, at the level of the first MCP joint. Insert the needle along this transmetacarpal line.
  - First dorsal: Radial side of the second metacarpal bone
  - Second dorsal: Radial side of the third metacarpal bone
  - Third dorsal: Ulnar side of the third metacarpal bone
  - Fourth dorsal: Ulnar side of the fourth metacarpal bone
- *Recommended Number of Injection Sites:* 1 site for each muscle

	Botox (units)	Dysport (units)	Xeomin (units)	Myobloc (units)
Suggested Dose	2.5–5[8]	10–20[8]	2.5–5[8]	100–500*

*Author recommendations.

(continued)

INJECTION PEARLS AND PITFALLS

For the first dorsal interosseous, if the needle is inserted too deeply, then it will be in the adductor pollicis. For the second dorsal interosseous, if the needle is inserted too deeply and radially, then it will be in the first volar interosseous or adductor pollicis. For the third dorsal interosseous, if the needle is too deep and ulnar, then it will be in the second volar interosseous. For the fourth dorsal interosseous, if the needle is inserted too deeply, then it will be in the third volar interosseous.

6.5 Palmar Interossei

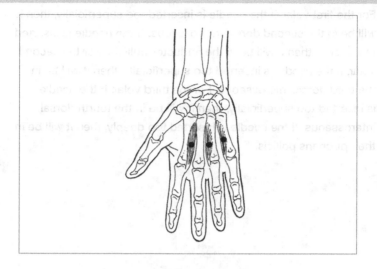

- *Muscle Origin:* Shaft of metacarpals of digits 2, 4, and 5
- *Muscle Insertion:* Extensor expansion of the finger of origin
- *Muscle Action:* Adduction of digits 2, 4, and 5; flexion at the MCP joints, extension of the IP joints
- *Injection Localization:* Draw a line perpendicular to the long axis of the hand, at the level of the first MCP joint. Insert the needle along this transmetacarpal line.
    - First volar: Ulnar side of the second metacarpal bone
    - Second volar: Radial side of the fourth metacarpal bone
    - Third volar: Radial side of the fifth metacarpal bone
- *Recommended Number of Injection Sites:* 1 site for each muscle

	Botox (units)	Dysport (units)	Xeomin (units)	Myobloc (units)
Suggested Dose	2.5–5[7,8]	10–20[8]	2.5–5[8]	100–500*

*Author recommendations.

(continued)

INJECTION PEARLS AND PITFALLS

For the first volar, if the needle is inserted too superficially, then it will be in the second dorsal interosseous. If the needle is inserted too deeply, then it will be in the adductor pollicis. For the second volar, if the needle is inserted too superficially, then it will be in the third dorsal interosseous. For the third volar, if the needle is inserted too superficially, then it will be in the fourth dorsal interosseous. If the needle is inserted too deeply, then it will be in the opponens pollicis.

6.6 Lumbricals

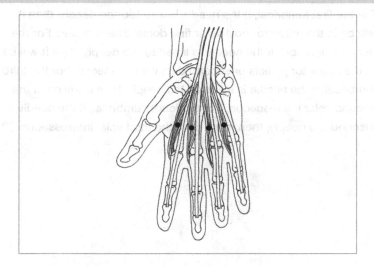

- *Muscle Origin:* Tendons of the flexor digitorum profundus
- *Muscle Insertion:* Radial portion of the extensor expansion of the proximal phalanges in digits 2 to 5
- *Muscle Action:* Extension of the IP joints; flexion of the MCP joints
- *Injection Localization:* Proximal to the MCP joint digits 2 to 4; radial to the flexor tendon
- *Recommended Number of Injection Sites:* 1 site for each muscle

	Botox (units)	Dysport (units)	Xeomin (units)	Myobloc (units)
Suggested Dose (per lumbrical)	2.5–15[2,6–8]	10–20[8]	2.5–10[8]	100–500*

*Author recommendations.

(*continued*)

INJECTION PEARLS AND PITFALLS

For the first lumbrical, if the needle is inserted too deeply, then it will be in the adductor pollicis or first dorsal interosseous. For the second lumbrical, if the needle is inserted too deeply, then it will be in the adductor pollicis or second dorsal interosseous. For the third lumbrical, if the needle is inserted too deeply, then it will be in the second volar interosseous. For the fourth lumbrical, if the needle is inserted too deeply, then it will be in the third volar interosseous.

References

1. Simpson DM, Patel AT, Alfaro A, et al. OnabotulinumtoxinA injection for poststroke upper-limb spasticity: guidance for early injectors from a Delphi panel process. *PM R*. 2017;9(2):136–148. doi:10.1016/j.pmrj.2016.06.016

2. Sheean G, Lannin NA, Turner-Stokes L, et al. Botulinum toxin assessment, intervention and after-care for upper limb hypertonicity in adults: international consensus statement. *Eur J Neurol*. 2010;17 (suppl 2):74–93. doi:10.1111/j.1468-1331.2010.03129.x

3. Ipsen. Dysport [package insert]. Published September 2019. https://www.ipsen.com/websites/Ipsen_Online/wp-content/uploads/sites/9/2020/01/09195739/S115_2019_09_25_sBLA_Approval_PMR_Fulfilled_PI_MG_Sept-2019.pdf

4. Merz. Xeomin [package insert]. Published August 2020. https://dailymed.nlm.nih.gov/dailymed/fda/fdaDrugXsl.cfm?setid=ccdc3aae-6e2d-4cd0-a51c-8375bfee9458&type=display

5. Pathak MS, Nguyen HT, Graham HK, Moore AP. Management of spasticity in adults: practical application of botulinum toxin. *Eur J Neurol*. 2006;13 (suppl 1):42–50. doi:10.1111/j.1468-1331.2006.01444.x

6. Francisco GE. Botulinum toxin: dosing and dilution. *Am J Phys Med Rehabil*. 2004;83(10 suppl):S30–S37. doi:10.1097/01.PHM.0000141128.62598.81

7. Nalysnyk L, Papapetropoulos S, Rotella P, et al. OnabotulinumtoxinA muscle injection patterns in adult spasticity: a systematic literature review. *BMC Neurol*. 2013;13:118. doi:10.1186/1471-2377-13-118

8. Jost W. *Pictorial Atlas of Botulinum Toxin Injection*. 2nd ed. Quintessence Publishing Co, Ltd; 2012.

9. Royal College of Physicians, British Society of Rehabilitation Medicine, Chartered Society of Physiotherapy, Association of Chartered Physiotherapists in Neurology and the Royal College of Occupational Therapists. Spasticity in adults: management using botulinum toxin. National guidelines. 2020. https://www.rcplondon.ac.uk/guidelines-policy/spasticity-adults-management-using-botulinum-toxin

10. Allergan. Botox [package insert]. Published July 2020. https://media.allergan.com/actavis/actavis/media/allergan-pdf-documents/product-prescribing/20190620-BOTOX-100-and-200-Units-v3-0USPI1145-v2-0MG1145.pdf

11. Kaňovský P, Slawek J, Denes Z, et al. Efficacy and safety of botulinum neurotoxin NT 201 in poststroke upper limb spasticity. *Clin Neuropharmacol*. 2009;32(5):259–265. doi:10.1097/WNF.0b013e3181b13308

12. Gracies JM, Bayle N, Goldberg S, Simpson DM. Botulinum toxin type B in the spastic arm: a randomized, double-blind, placebo-controlled, preliminary study. *Arch Phys Med Rehabil*. 2014;95(7):1303–1311. doi:10.1016/j.apmr.2014.03.016

PART III

Clinical Applications: Lower Limb Spasticity and Dystonia

CHAPTER 7

Muscles of the Pelvic Girdle and Hip

7.1 Iliopsoas

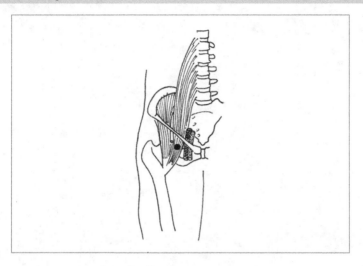

- *Muscle Origin:* Transverse processes and bodies of the lumbar vertebrae, iliac fossa
- *Muscle Insertion:* Lesser trochanter of the femur
- *Muscle Action:* Flexion and adduction at the hip
- *Injection Localization:* 2 fingerbreadths lateral to the femoral artery and 1 fingerbreadth distal to the inguinal ligament
- *Recommended Number of Injection Sites:* 1–3

	Botox® (units)	Dysport® (units)	Xeomin® (units)	Myobloc® (units)
Suggested Dose	25–200[1–5]	200–700[1,4,5]	25–200[4,5]	5,000–7,500[1]

(continued)

INJECTION PEARLS AND PITFALLS

If the needle is inserted too medially, then there is a risk of damaging the neurovascular bundle.

7.2 Gluteus Maximus

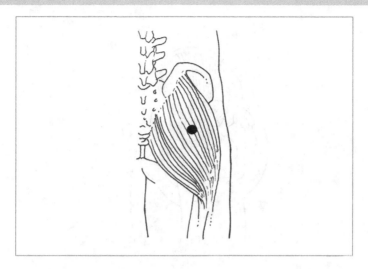

- *Muscle Origin:* Posterior surface ilium, sacroiliac and sacrotuberous ligaments, sacrum
- *Muscle Insertion:* Iliotibial tract, gluteal tuberosity of the femur
- *Muscle Action:* Extension, external rotation, and abduction at the hip
- *Injection Localization:* Midpoint of the line between the greater trochanter and the posterior superior iliac spine. Insert the needle until EMG activity is obtained.
- *Recommended Number of Injection Sites:* 1–3

	Botox (units)	Dysport (units)	Xeomin (units)	Myobloc (units)
Suggested Dose	40–100[4]	140–400[4]	40–100[4]	2,000–5,000*

*Author recommendations.

INJECTION PEARLS AND PITFALLS

Aim for the upper and outer quadrant of the buttock to avoid injecting the sciatic nerve.

7.3 Gluteus Medius

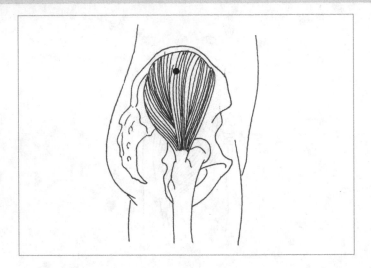

- *Muscle Origin:* Lateral surface of the ileum
- *Muscle Insertion:* Greater trochanter of the femur
- *Muscle Action:* The anterior fibers assist with abduction, internal rotation, and flexion at the hip. The posterior fibers assist with lateral rotation and extension at the hip.
- *Injection Localization:* One inch inferior to the midpoint of the iliac crest
- *Recommended Number of Injection Sites:* 1–2

	Botox (units)	Dysport (units)	Xeomin (units)	Myobloc (units)
Suggested Dose	20–100[4,5]	70–300[4,5]	20–100[4,5]	1,000–5,000*

*Author recommendations.

INJECTION PEARLS AND PITFALLS

If the needle is inserted too postero-medially, then it will be in the gluteus maximus. If the needle is inserted too antero-medially, then it will be in the tensor fasciae latae. If the needle is inserted too inferiorly, then it will be in the gluteus minimus or maximus.

7.4 Gluteus Minimus

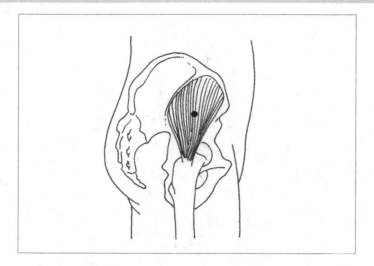

- *Muscle Origin:* Lateral surface of the ilium
- *Muscle Insertion:* Greater trochanter of the femur
- *Muscle Action:* Abduction, internal rotation, and flexion at the hip
- *Injection Localization:* Midway between the midpoint of the iliac crest and greater trochanter. Insert the needle down to the bone and retract slightly.
- *Recommended Number of Injection Sites:* 1–2

	Botox (units)	Dysport (units)	Xeomin (units)	Myobloc (units)
Suggested Dose	20–60[4]	70–200[4]	20–60[4]	1,000–3,000*

*Author recommendations.

INJECTION PEARLS AND PITFALLS

If the needle is inserted too superficially, then it will be in the gluteus medius.

7.5 Piriformis

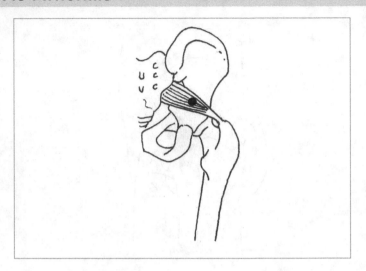

- *Muscle Origin:* Sacrum
- *Muscle Insertion:* Greater trochanter of femur
- *Muscle Action:* External rotation and abduction at the hip
- *Injection Localization:* Midpoint of a line between the posterior inferior iliac spine and greater trochanter, deep to the gluteus maximus
- *Recommended Number of Injection Sites:* 1–2

	Botox (units)	Dysport (units)	Xeomin (units)	Myobloc (units)
Suggested Dose	50–100[6–8]	150–300*	50–100[9]	2,000–4,000*

*Author recommendations.

INJECTION PEARLS AND PITFALLS

If the needle is inserted too superficially, then it will be in the gluteus maximus. If the needle is inserted too distally, then it will be in the hamstrings. Dosing recommendations for this muscle are adapted from literature regarding pain indications.

References

1. Pathak MS, Nguyen HT, Graham HK, Moore AP. Management of spasticity in adults: practical application of botulinum toxin. *Eur J Neurol*. 2006;13 (suppl 1):42–50. doi:10.1111/j.1468-1331.2006.01444.x

2. Nalysnyk L, Papapetropoulos S, Rotella P, et al. OnabotulinumtoxinA muscle injection patterns in adult spasticity: a systematic literature review. *BMC Neurol*. 2013;13:118. doi:10.1186/1471-2377-13-118

3. Esquenazi A, Alfaro A, Ayyoub Z, et al. OnabotulinumtoxinA for lower limb spasticity: guidance from a Delphi panel approach. *PM R*. 2017;9(10):960–968. doi:10.1016/j.pmrj.2017.02.014

4. Jost W. *Pictorial Atlas of Botulinum Toxin Injection*. 2nd ed. Quintessence Publishing Co, Ltd; 2012.

5. Royal College of Physicians, British Society of Rehabilitation Medicine, Chartered Society of Physiotherapy, Association of Chartered Physiotherapists in Neurology and the Royal College of Occupational Therapists. Spasticity in adults: management using botulinum toxin. National guidelines. 2020. https://www.rcplondon.ac.uk/guidelines -policy/spasticity-adults-management-using-botulinum-toxin

6. Fishman LM, Anderson C, Rosner B. BOTOX and physical therapy in the treatment of piriformis syndrome. *Am J Phys Med Rehabil*. 2002;81(12): 936–942. doi:10.1097/00002060-200212000-00009

7. Childers MK, Wilson DJ, Gnatz SM, et al. Botulinum toxin type A use in piriformis muscle syndrome: a pilot study. *Am J Phys Med Rehabil*. 2002;81(10):751–759. doi:10.1097/00002060-200210000-00006

8. Michel F, Decavel P, Toussirot E, et al. Piriformis muscle syndrome: diagnostic criteria and treatment of a monocentric series of 250 patients. *Ann Phys Rehabil Med*. 2013;56(5):371–383. doi:10.1016/j.rehab.2013.04.003

9. Rodriguez-Pinero M, Vidal Vargas V, Jimenez Sarmiento AS. Long-term efficacy of ultrasound-guided injection of incobotulinumtoxinA in piriformis syndrome. *Pain Med*. 2018;19(2):408–411. doi:10.1093/pm/pnx135

CHAPTER 8

Muscles of the Thigh

8.1 Adductor Magnus

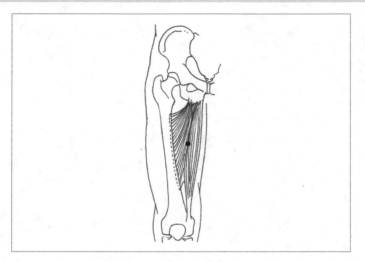

- *Muscle Origin:* Inferior ramus of the pubic, ischium, and ischial tuberosity
- *Muscle Insertion:* Anterior fibers—linea aspera. Posterior fibers—adductor tubercle of the femur
- *Muscle Action:* Adduction at the hip
- *Injection Localization:* Midpoint of the line between the medial femoral epicondyle and pubic tubercle
- *Recommended Number of Injection Sites:* 1–3

	Botox® (units)	Dysport® (units)	Xeomin® (units)	Myobloc® (units)
Suggested Dose	30–200[1–3]	100–500[3,4,]	30–150[3]	2,000–5000*

*Author recommendations.

(continued)

INJECTION PEARLS AND PITFALLS

If the needle is inserted too superficially, then it will be in the gracilis. If the needle is inserted too laterally, then it will be in the sartorius. If the needle is inserted too proximally, then it will be in the adductor longus.

8.2 Adductor Longus

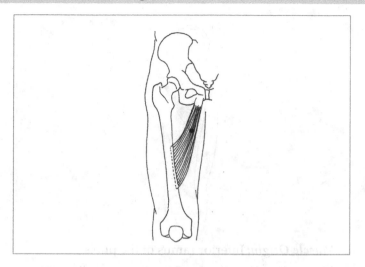

- *Muscle Origin:* Pubic tubercle
- *Muscle Insertion:* Medial lip of the linea aspera of the femur
- *Muscle Action:* Adduction and flexion at the hip
- *Injection Localization:* The tendon may be palpated arising from the pubic tubercle; insert the needle 4 finger-breadths distal to the pubic tubercle along the muscle belly
- *Recommended Number of Injection Sites:* 1–3

	Botox (units)	Dysport (units)	Xeomin (units)	Myobloc (units)
Suggested Dose	20–100[1–3]	50–400[3,4]	20–100[3]	1,500–3,000*

*Author recommendations.

INJECTION PEARLS AND PITFALLS

If the needle is inserted too deeply, then it will be in the adductor brevis. If the needle is too medial, then it will be in the gracilis. If the needle is inserted too laterally, then it will be in the sartorius. With proximal injection sites, diffusion into the bladder musculature may occur, which can lead to changes in bladder function.

8.3 Adductor Brevis

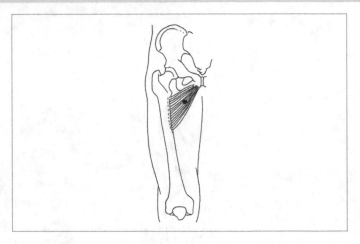

- **Muscle Origin:** Inferior ramus of the pubis
- **Muscle Insertion:** Pectineal line, proximal linea aspera of the femur
- **Muscle Action:** Adduction and flexion at the hip
- **Injection Localization:** The tendon may be palpated arising from the pubic tubercle; insert the needle 4 fingerbreadths distal to the pubic tubercle along the muscle belly, which will pierce the adductor longus.
- **Recommended Number of Injection Sites:** 1–2

	Botox (units)	Dysport (units)	Xeomin (units)	Myobloc (units)
Suggested Dose	20–100[1–3]	50–300[3,4]	20–80[3]	1,500–2,000*

*Author recommendations.

INJECTION PEARLS AND PITFALLS

If the needle is inserted too superficially and laterally, then it will be in the adductor longus. If the needle is inserted too superficially and medially, then it will be in the gracilis. If the needle is inserted too medially, then it will be in the adductor magnus. With proximal injection sites, diffusion into the bladder musculature may occur, which can lead to changes in bladder function.

8.4 Tensor Fasciae Latae

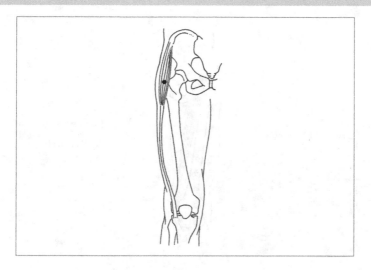

- *Muscle Origin:* Iliac crest posterior to the anterior superior iliac spine
- *Muscle Insertion:* Iliotibial tract
- *Muscle Action:* Flexion, internal rotation, and abduction at the hip
- *Injection Localization:* 2 fingerbreadths anterior to the greater trochanter
- *Recommended Number of Injection Sites:* 1–2

	Botox (units)	Dysport (units)	Xeomin (units)	Myobloc (units)
Suggested Dose	20–60[3]	80–300[3]	20–60[3]	1,000–2,500*

*Author recommendations.

INJECTION PEARLS AND PITFALLS

If the needle is inserted too anteriorly, then it will be in the sartorius or rectus femoris. If the needle is inserted too deeply, then it will be in the vastus lateralis. If the needle is inserted too posteriorly, then it will be in the gluteus medius.

8.5 Sartorius

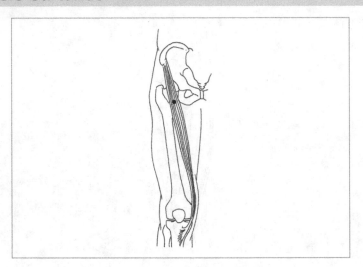

- *Muscle Origin:* Anterior superior iliac spine
- *Muscle Insertion:* Medial, proximal tibia at the pes anserinus
- *Muscle Action:* Primary function of the muscle includes flexion, abduction, and external rotation at the hip. Secondary action entails flexion at the knee.
- *Injection Localization:* 4 fingerbreadths distal to the anterior superior iliac spine along a line to the medial epicondyle of the tibia
- *Recommended Number of Injection Sites:* 1–2

	Botox (units)	Dysport (units)	Xeomin (units)	Myobloc (units)
Suggested Dose	10–40[3]	40–140[3]	10–40[3]	1,000–2,000*

*Author recommendations.

INJECTION PEARLS AND PITFALLS

If the needle is inserted too deeply or too distally, then it will be in the rectus femoris. If the needle is inserted too medially, there is a risk of hitting the femoral artery or being in the iliacus. If the needle is inserted too laterally, then it will be in the tensor fasciae latae.

8.6 Gracilis

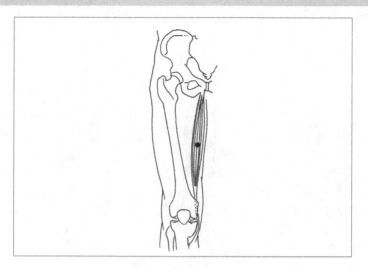

- *Muscle Origin:* Inferior ramus of the pubis and ramus of the ischium
- *Muscle Insertion:* Medial proximal tibia at the pes anserinus
- *Muscle Action:* Adduction of the thigh and flexion at the hip and knee; internal rotation at the hip
- *Injection Localization:* Midpoint between the pubic tubercle and medial femoral epicondyle
- *Recommended Number of Injection Sites:* 1–3

	Botox (units)	Dysport (units)	Xeomin (units)	Myobloc (units)
Suggested Dose	25–100[2,3,5]	75–300[3,5,]	25–100[3,5,]	1,250–3,000*

*Author recommendations.

INJECTION PEARLS AND PITFALLS

If the needle is inserted too deeply, then it will be in the adductor magnus. If the needle is inserted too laterally, then it will be in the adductor longus.

8.7 Rectus Femoris

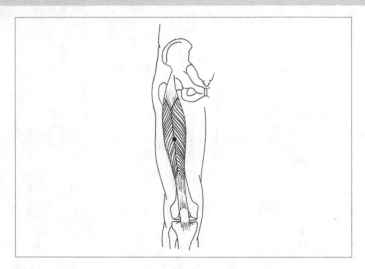

- *Muscle Origin:* Anterior inferior iliac spine, ilium
- *Muscle Insertion:* Patella and tibial tuberosity via patellar tendon
- *Muscle Action:* Extension of knee, flexion of hip
- *Injection Localization:* Midpoint of a line between the anterior superior iliac spine and the patella
- *Recommended Number of Injection Sites:* 1–3

	Botox (units)	Dysport (units)	Xeomin (units)	Myobloc (units)
Suggested Dose	20–150[1–3,5]	50–500[3,5]	20–100[3,5–7]	2,500–5,000*

*Author recommendations.

INJECTION PEARLS AND PITFALLS

If the needle is inserted too medially and too deeply, then it will be in the vastus intermedius. If the needle is inserted too laterally, then it will be in the vastus lateralis. If the needle is inserted too distally and medially, then it will be in the vastus medialis. For ambulatory patients, recommend initial conservative dosing.

8.8 Vastus Medialis

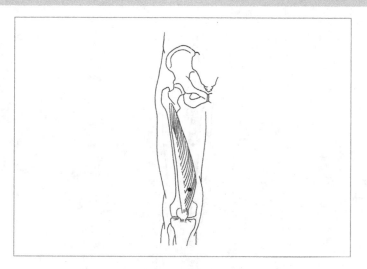

- *Muscle Origin:* Medial linea aspera of the femur, intertrochanteric line
- *Muscle Insertion:* Patella and tibial tuberosity via the patellar tendon
- *Muscle Action:* Extension of the knee
- *Injection Localization:* 4 fingerbreadths proximal to the medial angle of the patella
- *Recommended Number of Injection Sites:* 1–3

	Botox (units)	Dysport (units)	Xeomin (units)	Myobloc (units)
Suggested Dose	20–80[1–3]	50–300[3]	20–80[3,7]	1,000–3,000*

*Author recommendations.

INJECTION PEARLS AND PITFALLS

If the needle is inserted too posteriorly, then it will be in the sartorius or gracilis. If the needle is inserted anteriorly, then it will be in the rectus femoris. For ambulatory patients, recommend initial conservative dosing.

8.9 Vastus Intermedius

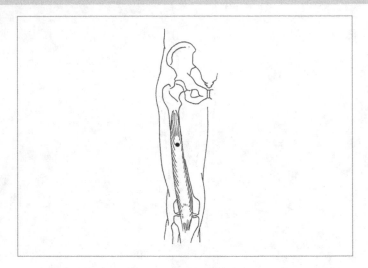

- ■ *Muscle Origin:* Anterior and lateral femur
- ■ *Muscle Insertion:* Patella and tibial tuberosity via the patellar tendon
- ■ *Muscle Action:* Extension of the knee
- ■ *Injection Localization:* Midpoint of a line between the patella and anterior superior iliac spine
- ■ *Recommended Number of Injection Sites:* 1–2

	Botox (units)	Dysport (units)	Xeomin (units)	Myobloc (units)
Suggested Dose	20–80[2,3]	50–300[3]	20–80[3]	1,000–3,000*

*Author recommendations.

INJECTION PEARLS AND PITFALLS

If the needle is inserted too superficially, then it will be in the rectus femoris. If the needle is inserted too laterally, then it will be in the vastus lateralis. If the needle is inserted too medially, then it will be in the vastus medialis or sartorius. For ambulatory patients, recommend initial conservative dosing.

8.10 Vastus Lateralis

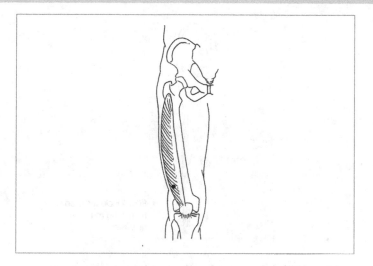

- **Muscle Origin:** Lateral linea aspera of the femur, intertrochanteric line
- **Muscle Insertion:** Patella and tibial tuberosity via the patellar tendon
- **Muscle Action:** Extension of the knee
- **Injection Localization:** 5 fingerbreadths proximal to the patella along the lateral aspect of the thigh
- **Recommended Number of Injection Sites:** 1–3

	Botox (units)	Dysport (units)	Xeomin (units)	Myobloc (units)
Suggested Dose	20–80[1-3]	50–300[3]	20–80[3]	1,000–3,000*

*Author recommendations.

INJECTION PEARLS AND PITFALLS

If the needle is inserted too medially, then it will be in the rectus femoris. For ambulatory patients, recommend initial conservative dosing.

8.11 Biceps Femoris (Long and Short Head)

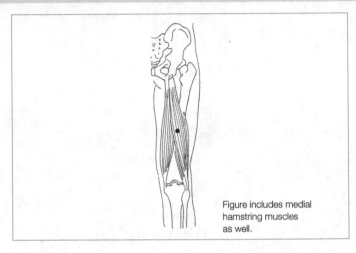

Figure includes medial hamstring muscles as well.

- *Muscle Origin:* Long head—ischial tuberosity; short head—linea aspera of femur
- *Muscle Insertion:* Head of the fibula; lateral condyle of the tibia
- *Muscle Action:* Extension and external rotation at the hip; flexion at the knee
- *Injection Localization:* Midpoint of a line between the fibular head and ischial tuberosity
- *Recommended Number of Injection Sites:* 1–3

	Botox (units)	Dysport (units)	Xeomin (units)	Myobloc (units)
Suggested Dose	30–150[1–3,5,8]	100–400[3,5,8]	40–150[3,5–7]	1,500–5,000*

*Author recommendations.

INJECTION PEARLS AND PITFALLS

If the needle is inserted too medially, then it will be in the semimembranosus.

8.12 Semimembranosus

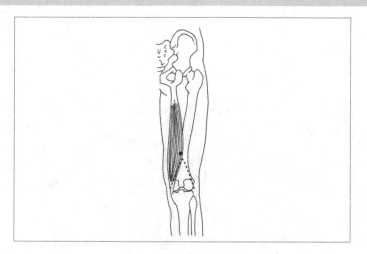

- **_Muscle Origin:_** Ischial tuberosity

- **_Muscle Insertion:_** Medial condyle of the tibia

- **_Muscle Action:_** Extension and internal rotation at the hip; flexion at the knee

- **_Injection Localization:_** Locate the apex of the "V" in the posterior leg with the border of the "V" being the semitendinosus (medial) and biceps femoris (lateral) tendons. The semimembranosus is lateral to the semitendinosus tendon in the apex of the "V."

- **_Recommended Number of Injection Sites:_** 1–3

	Botox (units)	Dysport (units)	Xeomin (units)	Myobloc (units)
Suggested Dose	20–150[1,3,5]	80–400[3,5,8]	20–150[3,5]	1,500–5,000*

*Author recommendations.

INJECTION PEARLS AND PITFALLS

If the needle is inserted too medially, then it will be in the semitendinosus. If the needle is inserted too laterally, then it will be in the biceps femoris or sciatic nerve. If the needle is inserted too deeply, then it will be in the adductor magnus.

8.13 Semitendinosus

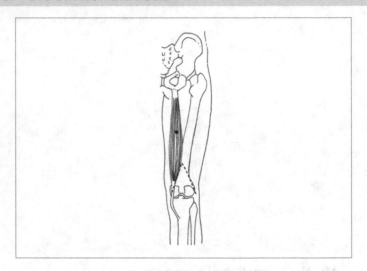

- *Muscle Origin:* Ischial tuberosity
- *Muscle Insertion:* Medial proximal tibia at the pes anserinus
- *Muscle Action:* Extension and internal rotation at the hip; flexion at the knee
- *Injection Localization:* Midpoint of a line between the medial epicondyle of the femur and the ischial tuberosity
- *Recommended Number of Injection Sites:* 1–3

	Botox (units)	Dysport (units)	Xeomin (units)	Myobloc (units)
Suggested Dose	20–150[1,3,5]	80–400[3,5,8]	20–150[3,5]	1,500–5,000*

*Author recommendations.

INJECTION PEARLS AND PITFALLS

If the needle is inserted too laterally, then it will be in the semimembranosus or biceps femoris. If the needle is inserted too medially or too deeply, then it will be in the semimembranosus.

References

1. Nalysnyk L, Papapetropoulos S, Rotella P, et al. OnabotulinumtoxinA muscle injection patterns in adult spasticity: a systematic literature review. *BMC Neurol.* 2013;13:118. doi:10.1186/1471-2377-13-118
2. Esquenazi A, Alfaro A, Ayyoub Z, et al. OnabotulinumtoxinA for lower limb spasticity: guidance from a Delphi panel approach. *PM R.* 2017;9(10):960–968. doi:10.1016/j.pmrj.2017.02.014
3. Jost W. *Pictorial Atlas of Botulinum Toxin Injection.* 2nd ed. Quintessence Publishing Co, Ltd; 2012.
4. Hyman N, Barnes M, Bhakta B, et al. Botulinum toxin (Dysport) treatment of hip adductor spasticity in multiple sclerosis: a prospective, randomised, double blind, placebo controlled, dose ranging study. *J Neurol Neurosurg Psychiatry.* 2000;68(6):707–712. doi:10.1136/jnnp.68.6.707
5. Royal College of Physicians, British Society of Rehabilitation Medicine, Chartered Society of Physiotherapy, Association of Chartered Physiotherapists in Neurology and the Royal College of Occupational Therapists. Spasticity in adults: management using botulinum toxin. National guidelines. 2020. https://www.rcplondon.ac.uk/guidelines -policy/spasticity-adults-management-using-botulinum-toxin
6. Santamato A, Panza F, Ranieri M, et al. Efficacy and safety of higher doses of botulinum toxin type A NT 201 free from complexing proteins in the upper and lower limb spasticity after stroke. *J Neural Transm (Vienna).* 2013;120(3):469–476. doi:10.1007/s00702-012-0892-x
7. Intiso D, Simone V, Di Rienzo F, et al. High doses of a new botulinum toxin type A (NT-201) in adult patients with severe spasticity following brain injury and cerebral palsy. *NeuroRehabilitation.* 2014;34(3):515–522. doi:10.3233/NRE-141052
8. Olver J, Esquenazi A, Fung VS, et al. Botulinum toxin assessment, intervention and aftercare for lower limb disorders of movement and muscle tone in adults: international consensus statement. *Eur J Neurol.* 2010;17 (suppl 2):57–73. doi:10.1111/j.1468-1331.2010.03128.x

CHAPTER 9

Muscles of the Lower Leg

9.1 Gastrocnemius

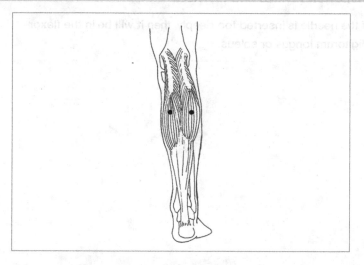

- *Muscle Origin:* Posterior surface of the femur proximal to the medial and lateral femoral condyles
- *Muscle Insertion:* Calcaneus through the Achilles tendon
- *Muscle Action:* Ankle plantar flexion; flexion at the knee
- *Injection Localization:* Medial/Lateral heads: 5 finger-breadths distal to the popliteal crease along the medial or lateral aspect of the calf, respectively
- *Recommended Number of Injection Sites:* 1–3 per head

(continued)

	Botox® (units)	Dysport® (units)	Xeomin® (units)	Myobloc® (units)
Suggested Dose (per head)	20–100[1-6] (75)[†,7]	80–200[2,4-6] (100–150)[†,8]	20–100[5,6,9,10]	1,000–3,000*

[†]Denotes FDA-approved dosing.

*Author recommendations.

INJECTION PEARLS AND PITFALLS

If the needle is inserted too deeply, then it will be in the flexor digitorum longus or soleus.

9.2 Soleus

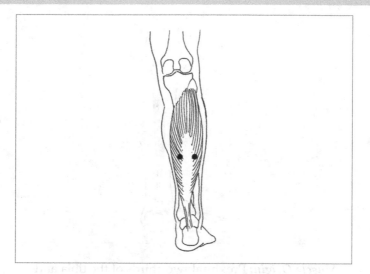

- *Muscle Origin:* Popliteal line, proximal tibia and fibula
- *Muscle Insertion:* Calcaneus through the Achilles tendon
- *Muscle Action:* Ankle plantar flexion
- *Injection Localization:* Distal to the belly of the gastrocnemius muscle, avoiding the Achilles tendon
- *Recommended Number of Injection Sites:* 1–3

	Botox (units)	Dysport (units)	Xeomin (units)	Myobloc (units)
Suggested Dose	20–150[1–3,5,6] (75)[†,7]	80–500[2,4–6] (330–500)[†,8]	20–100[5,6,9,10]	2,500–5,000*

[†]Denotes FDA-approved dosing.

*Author recommendations.

INJECTION PEARLS AND PITFALLS

Stay above the mid-calf to minimize the risk of injecting the tendinous area. If the needle is inserted too superficially, then it will be in the gastrocnemius.

9.3 Tibialis Posterior

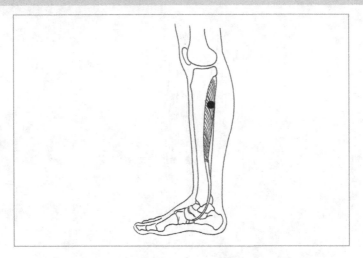

- *Muscle Origin:* Proximal two-thirds of the tibia and fibula, interosseous membrane
- *Muscle Insertion:* Navicular cuneiform cuboid, and bases of the second and fourth metatarsal
- *Muscle Action:* Adduct the front of the foot; inversion and plantar flexion at the ankle
- *Injection Localization:* 4 fingerbreadths distal to the tibial tuberosity and 1 fingerbreadth off the medial edge of the tibia directed posterior to the tibia. The needle will pass through the soleus and flexor digitorum longus muscles.
- *Recommended Number of Injection Sites:* 1–3

	Botox (units)	Dysport (units)	Xeomin (units)	Myobloc (units)
Suggested Dose	25–100[1,2,11] (75)[†,12]	100–300[4] (200–300)[†,13]	20–100[5,6]	2,500–5,000[11]

[†]Denotes FDA-approved dosing.

INJECTION PEARLS AND PITFALLS

If the needle is inserted too superficially, then it will be in the soleus or flexor digitorum longus.

9.4 Tibialis Anterior

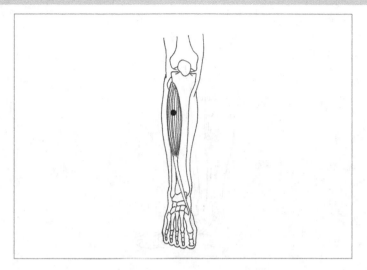

- *Muscle Origin:* Lateral condyle of the tibia, proximal two-thirds of the lateral surface of the tibia, interosseous membrane, and deep fascia of the leg
- *Muscle Insertion:* Medial cuneiform, base of first metatarsal
- *Muscle Action:* Inversion and dorsiflexion of the foot
- *Injection Localization:* 4 fingerbreadths below the tibial tuberosity and 1 fingerbreadth lateral to the tibial crest
- *Recommended Number of Injection Sites:* 1–3

	Botox (units)	Dysport (units)	Xeomin (units)	Myobloc (units)
Suggested Dose	25–75[2,11]	75–300[4,6,11]	20–75[5,6]	1,000–2,500[11]

INJECTION PEARLS AND PITFALLS

If the needle is inserted too laterally and too deeply, then it will be in the extensor digitorum longus.

9.5 Peroneus Longus

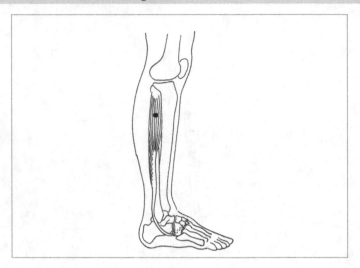

- *Muscle Origin:* Proximal two-thirds of the lateral surface of the fibula

- *Muscle Insertion:* Base of the first metatarsal, medial cuneiform

- *Muscle Action:* Eversion and weak plantar flexion at the ankle

- *Injection Localization:* 3 fingerbreadths distal to the fibular head along the lateral surface of the leg. The needle is directed toward the lateral aspect of the fibula.

- *Recommended Number of Injection Sites:* 1

	Botox (units)	Dysport (units)	Xeomin (units)	Myobloc (units)
Suggested Dose	25–80[4,5]	100–250[4]	50–80[5]	1,250–3,000*

*Author recommendations.

INJECTION PEARLS AND PITFALLS

If the needle is inserted too posteriorly, then it will be in the soleus. If the needle is inserted too anteriorly, it will be in the extensor digitorum longus.

9.6 Peroneus Brevis

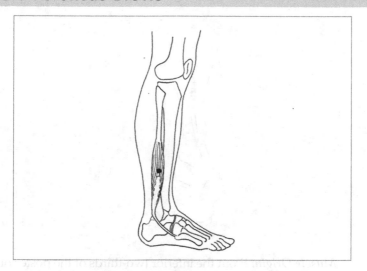

- *Muscle Origin:* Distal two-thirds of the lateral surface of the fibula, adjacent to the intermuscular septa

- *Muscle Insertion:* Dorsal surface of the base of the fifth metatarsal

- *Muscle Action:* Eversion and weak plantar flexion at the ankle

- *Injection Localization:* 1 handbreadth proximal to the lateral malleolus and anterior to the peroneus longus tendon

- *Recommended Number of Injection Sites:* 1

	Botox (units)	Dysport (units)	Xeomin (units)	Myobloc (units)
Suggested Dose	30–40[5]	80–120[4]	30–40[5]	1,500–2,000*

*Author recommendations.

INJECTION PITFALLS

If the needle is inserted too superficially, then it will be in the soleus. If the needle is inserted too deeply, then it will be in the tibialis posterior.

9.7 Flexor Hallucis Longus

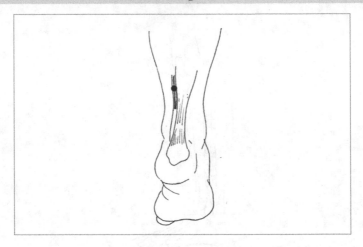

- *Muscle Origin:* From the inferior two-thirds of the posterior surface of the body of the fibula and interosseous membrane
- *Muscle Insertion:* Into the base of the distal phalanx of the great toe
- *Muscle Action:* Flexes great toe
- *Injection Localization:* Insert the needle 5 fingerbreadths above the insertion of the Achilles tendon and medial border of the tibia.
- *Recommended Number of Injection Sites:* 1–2

	Botox (units)	Dysport (units)	Xeomin (units)	Myobloc (units)
Suggested Dose	25–75[4,14] (50)[†,12]	70–200[†,13]	40–60[5,6]	1,500–3,500[14]

†Denotes FDA-approved dosing.

INJECTION PEARLS AND PITFALLS

If the needle is inserted too deeply, it will be in the posterior tibialis. If the needle is inserted too anteriorly, it will be in the flexor digitorum longus. If the needle is inserted too proximal, it will be in the lower fibers of the soleus.

9.8 Flexor Digitorum Longus

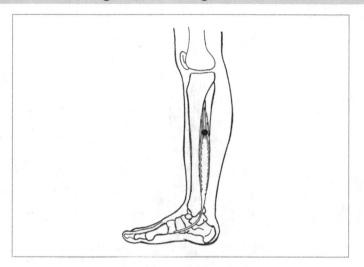

- *Muscle Origin:* Posterior surface of the tibia
- *Muscle Insertion:* Bases of the distal phalanges of the second to fifth toes
- *Muscle Action:* Flexes the toes without plantarflexing the ankle
- *Injection Localization:* In the middle of the tibial shaft, 1 fingerbreadth posterior to the medial margin
- *Recommended Number of Injection Sites:* 1

	Botox (units)	Dysport (units)	Xeomin (units)	Myobloc (units)
Suggested Dose	25–100[1,4,14,15] (50)[†,12]	130–200[†,13]	40–60[5]	1,250–5,000*

†Denotes FDA-approved dosing.

*Author recommendations.

INJECTION PEARLS AND PITFALLS

If the needle is inserted too superficially, then it will be in the soleus. If the needle is inserted too deeply, then it will be in the tibialis posterior.

9.9 Extensor Hallucis Longus

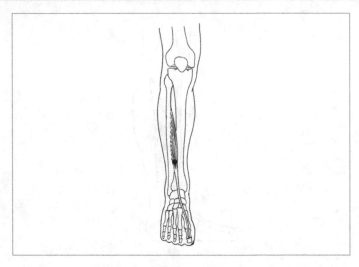

- *Muscle Origin:* Midportion of the shaft of the fibula
- *Muscle Insertion:* Distal phalanx of the great toe
- *Muscle Action:* Extends the great toe and dorsiflexes the ankle
- *Injection Localization:* 3 fingerbreadths above the bimalleolar line of the ankle just lateral to the crest of the tibia
- *Recommended Number of Injection Sites:* 1

	Botox (units)	Dysport (units)	Xeomin (units)	Myobloc (units)
Suggested Dose	20–60[5,6]	75–200[11]	20–60[5,6]	1,000–3,000*

*Author recommendations.

INJECTION PEARLS AND PITFALLS

If the needle is inserted too superficially and too proximally, then it will be in the tibialis anterior. If the needle is inserted too laterally, then it will be in the peroneus tertius.

9.10 Extensor Digitorum Longus

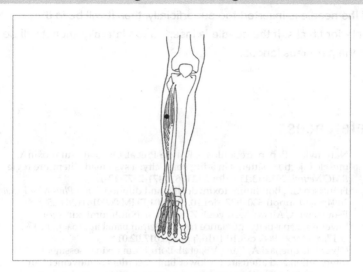

- *Muscle Origin:* Proximal, lateral condyle of the tibia; proximal three-fourths of the anterior surface of the fibula, interosseous membrane, and crural fascia

- *Muscle Insertion:* Middle and distal phalanges of the lateral 4 toes

- *Muscle Action:* Extension of the lateral 4 toes; dorsiflexion and eversion at the ankle

- *Injection Localization:* 4 fingerbreadths distal to the tibial tubercle and 2 fingerbreadths lateral to the tibial crest. The needle is inserted through the anterior tibialis muscle.

- *Recommended Number of Injection Sites:* 1

	Botox (units)	Dysport (units)	Xeomin (units)	Myobloc (units)
Suggested Dose	25–75*	75–200*	25–75*	1,250–3,500*

*Author recommendations.

(continued)

INJECTION PEARLS AND PITFALLS

If the needle is inserted too superficially, then it will be in the anterior tibialis. If the needle is inserted too laterally, then it will be in the peroneus longus.

References

1.   Nalysnyk L, Papapetropoulos S, Rotella P, et al. OnabotulinumtoxinA muscle injection patterns in adult spasticity: a systematic literature review. *BMC Neurol.* 2013;13:118. doi:10.1186/1471-2377-13-118

2.   Francisco GE. Botulinum toxin: dosing and dilution. *Am J Phys Med Rehabil.* 2004;83(10 suppl):S30–S37. doi:10.1097/01.PHM.0000141128.62598.81

3.   Esquenazi A, Alfaro A, Ayyoub Z, et al. OnabotulinumtoxinA for lower limb spasticity: guidance from a Delphi panel approach. *PM R.* 2017;9(10):960–968. doi:10.1016/j.pmrj.2017.02.014

4.   Olver J, Esquenazi A, Fung VS, et al. Botulinum toxin assessment, intervention and aftercare for lower limb disorders of movement and muscle tone in adults: international consensus statement. *Eur J Neurol.* 2010;17 (suppl 2):57–73. doi:10.1111/j.1468-1331.2010.03128.x

5.   Royal College of Physicians, British Society of Rehabilitation Medicine Chartered Society of Physiotherapy, Association of Chartered Physiotherapists in Neurology and the Royal College of Occupational Therapists. Spasticity in adults: management using botulinum toxin. National guidelines. RCP. Published 2018. https://www.rcplondon.ac.uk/guidelines-policy/spasticity-adults-management-using-botulinum-toxin

6.   Jost W. *Pictorial Atlas of Botulinum Toxin Injection.* 2nd ed. Quintessence Publishing Co, Ltd; 2012.

7.   Allergan. Botox [Package insert]. Published July 2020. https://media.allergan.com/actavis/actavis/media/allergan-pdf-documents/product-prescribing/20190620-BOTOX-100-and-200-Units-v3-0USPI1145-v2-0MG1145.pdf

8.   Ipsen. Dysport [package insert]. Published September 2019. https://www.ipsen.com/websites/Ipsen_Online/wp-content/uploads/sites/9/2020/01/09195739/S115_2019_09_25_sBLA_Approval_PMR_Fulfilled_PI_MG_Sept-2019.pdf

9.   Santamato A, Panza F, Ranieri M, et al. Efficacy and safety of higher doses of botulinum toxin type A NT 201 free from complexing proteins in the upper and lower limb spasticity after stroke. *J Neural Transm (Vienna).* 2013;120(3):469–476. doi:10.1007/s00702-012-0892-x

10. Intiso D, Simone V, Di Rienzo F, et al. High doses of a new botulinum toxin type A (NT-201) in adult patients with severe spasticity following brain injury and cerebral palsy. *NeuroRehabilitation.* 2014;34(3):515–522. doi:10.3233/NRE-141052

11. Pathak MS, Nguyen HT, Graham HK, Moore AP. Management of spasticity in adults: practical application of botulinum toxin. *Eur J Neurol.* 2006;13 (suppl 1):42–50. doi:10.1111/j.1468-1331.2006.01444.x

12. Allergan. Botox [package insert]. Published July 2020. https://media
    .allergan.com/actavis/actavis/media/allergan-pdf-documents/product
    -prescribing/20190620-BOTOX-100-and-200-Units-v3-0USPI1145-v2
    -0MG1145.pdf
13. Ipsen. Dysport [package insert]. Published September 2019. https://
    www.ipsen.com/websites/Ipsen_Online/wp-content/uploads/
    sites/9/2020/01/09195739/S115_2019_09_25_sBLA_Approval_PMR
    _Fulfilled_PI_MG_Sept-2019.pdf
14. Charles D, Gill CE. Neurotoxin injection for movement disorders.
    Continuum (Minneap Minn). 2010;16(1 Movement Disorders):131–157.
    doi:10.1212/01.CON.0000348904.32834.70
15. Wissel J, Ward AB, Erztgaard P, et al. European consensus table on the use
    of botulinum toxin type A in adult spasticity. *J Rehabil Med*. 2009;41(1):
    13–25. doi:10.2340/16501977-0303

CHAPTER 10

Muscles of the Foot

10.1 Flexor Hallucis Brevis

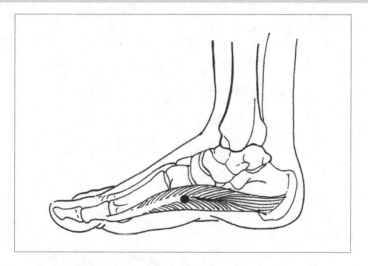

- *Muscle Origin:* Cuboid bone, lateral cuneiform and tendon of the tibialis posterior muscle
- *Muscle Insertion:* Medial and lateral sides of the proximal phalanx of the great toe
- *Muscle Action:* Flexion of the proximal phalanx of the great toe
- *Injection Localization:* 3–4 fingerbreadths proximal to the head of the first metatarsal, medial to the flexor hallucis longus tendon
- *Recommended Number of Injection Sites:* 1

	Botox® (units)	Dysport® (units)	Xeomin® (units)	Myobloc® (units)
Suggested Dose	10–30[1–3]	20–100[1,2]	10–30[1,2]	250–1,000*

*Author recommendations.

(continued)

INJECTION PEARLS AND PITFALLS

If the needle is inserted too laterally, then it will be in the adductor hallucis. If the needle is inserted too medially, then it will be in the abductor hallucis.

10.2 Flexor Digitorum Brevis

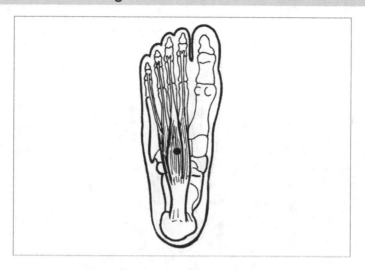

- *Muscle Origin:* Medial process of the calcaneal tuberosity; medial and lateral intermuscular septa
- *Muscle Insertion:* Middle phalanges of the lateral 4 toes
- *Muscle Action:* Flexion of the middle phalanges of the 4 lateral toes
- *Injection Localization:* Midway between the third metatarsal head and the calcaneus
- *Recommended Number of Injection Sites:* 1

	Botox (units)	Dysport (units)	Xeomin (units)	Myobloc (units)
Suggested Dose	10–40[2,4,5]	30–80[2,4]	10–20[2]	250–1,000*

*Author recommendations.

INJECTION PEARLS AND PITFALLS

If the needle is inserted too laterally, then it will be in the abductor digiti minimi. If the needle is inserted too medially, then it will be in the abductor hallucis brevis. If the needle is inserted too deeply, then it will be in the quadratus plantae.

10.3 Adductor Hallucis

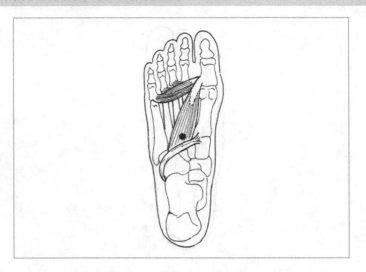

- *Muscle Origin:* Oblique head—bases of the second to fourth metatarsals, sheath of peroneus longus tendon; transverse head—capsules of the third to fifth metatarsal-phalangeal joints, associated deep transverse metatarsal ligaments

- *Muscle Insertion:* Base of the proximal phalanx of the great toe

- *Muscle Action:* Adduction and flexion of the great toe

- *Injection Localization:* 1 fingerbreadth below the navicular bone on the mid-portion of the medial aspect of the foot. Oblique head is commonly injected.

- *Recommended Number of Injection Sites:* 1

	Botox (units)	Dysport (units)	Xeomin (units)	Myobloc (units)
Suggested Dose	5–20[1]	20–80[1]	5–20[1]	250–1,000*

*Author recommendations.

INJECTION PEARLS AND PITFALLS

If the needle is inserted too superficially, then it will be in the lumbricals.

10.4 Quadratus Plantae

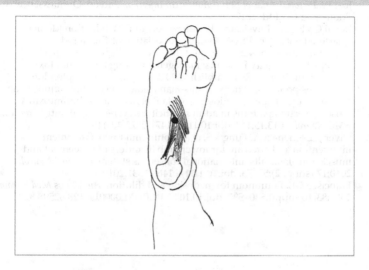

- *Muscle Origin:* Medial and lateral side of the plantar surface of the calcaneus

- *Muscle Insertion:* Lateral and posterior margin of the flexor digitorum longus tendon

- *Muscle Action:* Aids in flexion of the lateral 4 toes by modifying the pull of the flexor digitorum longus tendon

- *Injection Localization:* Midway in a line between the calcaneal tuberosity and the head of the third metatarsal. Insert until the resistance of the lateral cuneiform can be felt, then retract the needle slightly.

- *Recommended Number of Injection Sites:* 1

	Botox (units)	Dysport (units)	Xeomin (units)	Myobloc (units)
Suggested Dose	5–20[1]	20–80[1]	5–20[1]	250–1,000*

*Author recommendations.

INJECTION PEARLS AND PITFALLS

If the needle is inserted too superficially, then it will be in the flexor digitorum brevis. If the needle is injected too laterally, then it will be in the abductor digiti minimi.

References

1. Jost W. *Pictorial Atlas of Botulinum Toxin Injection*. 2nd ed. Quintessence Publishing Co, Ltd; 2012.
2. Royal College of Physicians, British Society of Rehabilitation Medicine, Chartered Society of Physiotherapy, Association of Chartered Physiotherapists in Neurology and the Royal College of Occupational Therapists. Spasticity in adults: management using botulinum toxin. National guidelines. RCP. Published 2018. https://www.rcplondon.ac.uk/guidelines-policy/spasticity-adults-management-using-botulinum-toxin
3. Nalysnyk L, Papapetropoulos S, Rotella P, et al. OnabotulinumtoxinA muscle injection patterns in adult spasticity: a systematic literature review. *BMC Neurol*. 2013;13:118. doi:10.1186/1471-2377-13-118
4. Olver J, Esquenazi A, Fung VS, et al. Botulinum toxin assessment, intervention and aftercare for lower limb disorders of movement and muscle tone in adults: international consensus statement. *Eur J Neurol*. 2010;17 (suppl 2):57–73. doi:10.1111/j.1468-1331.2010.03128.x
5. Francisco GE. Botulinum toxin: dosing and dilution. *Am J Phys Med Rehabil*. 2004;83(10 suppl):S30–S37. doi:10.1097/01.PHM.0000141128.62598.81

Clinical Applications: Axial Spasticity and Dystonia

PART TWO

Clinical Applications: Axial
Spasticity and Dystonia

CHAPTER 11

Muscles of the Head

11.1 Frontalis

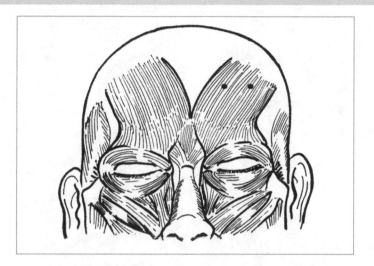

- *Muscle Origin:* Anterior portion of the galea aponeurotica
- *Muscle Insertion:* Fibers of the orbicularis oculi and procerus
- *Muscle Action:* Elevation of the eyebrows, wrinkling the forehead skin
- *Injection Localization:* Localization may be altered based on the indication. For migraine, inject in the upper-third of the forehead.
- *Recommended Number of Injection Sites:* 1–3 on each side

	Botox® (units)	Dysport® (units)	Xeomin® (units)	Myobloc® (units)
Suggested Dose per side	2.5–10[1] (10)[†,2,3]	15–60[1]	2.5–10[1]	125–1,000*

*Author recommendations.

[†]Denotes FDA-approved dosing.

(*continued*)

INJECTION PEARLS AND PITFALLS

If the needle hits the skull, withdraw until it is in the muscle belly. It is recommended that the needle be inserted in a way that the tip will be away from the midline. The needle should be inserted at a 45-degree angle superiorly and superficial to the corrugator muscle to minimize the spread. Avoid injection in the low, lateral forehead to minimize ptosis.

11.2 Procerus

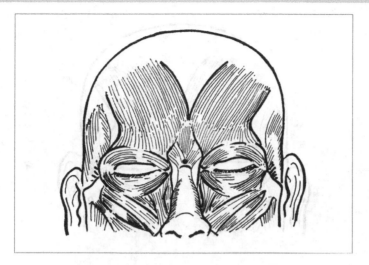

- *Muscle Origin:* Nasal bone and lateral nasal cartilage
- *Muscle Insertion:* Skin between the eyebrows
- *Muscle Action:* Draws down the middle part of the eyebrows
- *Injection Localization:* Midline into the belly of the muscle between the furrowed brows
- *Recommended Number of Injection Sites:* 1

	Botox (units)	Dysport (units)	Xeomin (units)	Myobloc (units)
Suggested Dose	2.5–5[1]	10–20[1]	2.5–5[1]	125–250*
	(4–5)[†,2,3]	(10)[†,4]	(4)[†,5]	

*Author recommendations.

[†]Denotes FDA-approved dosing.

INJECTION PEARLS AND PITFALLS

If the needle is inserted too laterally, then it will be in the orbicularis oculi.

11.3 Corrugator

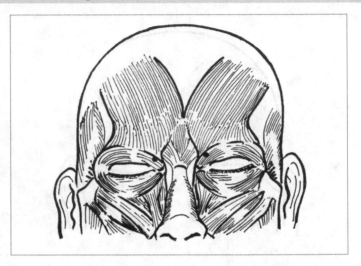

- *Muscle Origin:* Nasal portion of the frontal bone
- *Muscle Insertion:* Medial third of the eyebrow skin, epicranial aponeurosis
- *Muscle Action:* Draws down the middle part of the eyebrow, causing deep frown lines
- *Injection Localization:* Furrow the eyebrow and grasp the muscle belly over the medial edge of the eyebrow.
- *Recommended Number of Injection Sites:* 1–2 each side

	Botox (units)	Dysport (units)	Xeomin (units)	Myobloc (units)
Suggested Dose	2.5–5[1] (4–5)[†,2,3]	10–20[1] (10)[†,4]	2.5–5[1] (4)[†,5]	125–250*

*Author recommendations.

[†]Denotes FDA-approved dosing.

INJECTION PEARLS AND PITFALLS

There is an increased risk of ptosis if the needle is injected too deeply and medially. The needle should be inserted at a 90-degree angle with the bevel of the needle pointing superiorly into the muscle belly.

11.4 Orbicularis Oculi

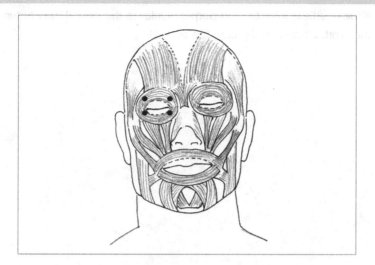

- *Muscle Origin:* Circumferential muscle with multiple origin points, including the front surface of the orbital margin

- *Muscle Insertion:* Lateral palpebral raphe

- *Muscle Action:* Closes the eyelids

- *Injection Localization:* For the lower medial site, pinch the lower lid and inject subcutaneously, directing the needle nasally. For the lower lateral site, pinch the lateral lower lid and inject subcutaneously, directing the needle temporally. For the upper lateral site, pinch the upper lateral eyelid and inject subcutaneously, directing the needle toward the earlobe. For the upper medial site, pinch the upper medial eyelid and direct the needle nasally.

- *Recommended Number of Injection Sites:* 3–5

	Botox (units)	Dysport (units)	Xeomin (units)	Myobloc (units)
Suggested Dose	5–20[1] (3.75–12)[†,2,3]	20–80[1]	5–20[1] (4–8)[†,5]	250–1,000*

*Author recommendations.

[†]Denotes FDA-approved dosing.

(continued)

INJECTION PEARLS AND PITFALLS

If the needle is inserted too perpendicular to the skin, it may enter the orbit, which can damage the eyeball.

11.5 Nasalis

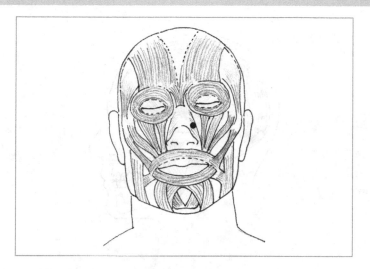

- *Muscle Origin:* Middle of the maxilla; alar part—alveolar yoke of the second incisor; transverse part—alveolar yoke of the canine

- *Muscle Insertion:* Alar part—ala of the nose, margin of the nostrils; transverse part—lateral nasal cartilage, dorsal aponeurosis of the nose

- *Muscle Action:* Alar part widens the nasal openings and flares the nostrils. Transverse part narrows the nares and lowers the tip of the nose.

- *Injection Localization:* Side of the nose, superficially

- *Recommended Number of Injection Sites:* 1–2 each side

	Botox (units)	Dysport (units)	Xeomin (units)	Myobloc (units)
Suggested Dose	2.5–5[1,6]	10–20[1]	2.5–5[1]	125–250*

*Author recommendations.

INJECTION PEARLS AND PITFALLS

If the needle is inserted too laterally, then the needle will be in the levator labii superioris alaeque nasi.

11.6 Temporalis

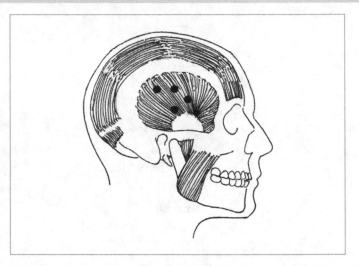

- *Muscle Origin:* Lateral surface of the skull, temporal fossa
- *Muscle Insertion:* Coronoid process and anterior, medial part of the ramus of the mandible
- *Muscle Action:* The anterior fibers assist in elevation of the mandible; posterior fibers assist in retrusion of the mandible.
- *Injection Localization:* Site 1: 2 fingerbreadths superior to the tragus. Site 2: 2 fingerbreadths superior to Site 1. Site 3: 1 fingerbreadth anterior and inferior to Site 2. Site 4: 1 fingerbreadth posterior to Site 2.
- *Recommended Number of Injection Sites:* 1–4

	Botox (units)	Dysport (units)	Xeomin (units)	Myobloc (units)
Suggested Dose	5–40[1] (20)[†,2]	20–160[1]	5–40[1]	250–1,000*

*Author recommendations.

†Denotes FDA-approved dosing.

(*continued*)

INJECTION PEARLS AND PITFALLS

If the needle is inserted too closely to the external eye orbit, then it will be in the orbicularis oculi. If the needle is inserted too closely to the zygomatic arch, then the needle will be in the tendinous portion of the temporal muscle.

11.7 Masseter

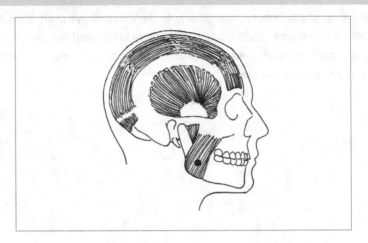

- *Muscle Origin:* Zygomatic arch
- *Muscle Insertion:* Ramus and lateral surface of the angle of the mandible
- *Muscle Action:* Elevation and protrusion of the mandible
- *Injection Localization:* One fingerbreadth posterior to the anterior edge of the muscle and 1 fingerbreadth cephalad to the lower edge of the mandible
- *Recommended Number of Injection Sites:* 1–3

	Botox (units)	Dysport (units)	Xeomin (units)	Myobloc (units)
Suggested Dose	5–45[1,7]	20–180[1]	5–45[1]	250–2,000*

*Author recommendations.

INJECTION PEARLS AND PITFALLS

The anterior edge is recognizable when the patient clenches his teeth. If the needle is inserted too close to the zygomatic arch, the duct of the parotid gland can be damaged. If the needle is inserted too posteriorly, then it will go through the parotid gland. If the needle is inserted too anteriorly, then the tip may end up in the oral cavity.

11.8 Lateral Pterygoid

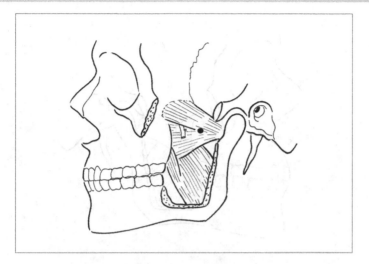

- *Muscle Origin:* Inferior head—lateral surface of the lateral pterygoid plate of the sphenoid bone. Superior head—greater wing of the sphenoid bone

- *Muscle Insertion:* Superior head—temporomandibular joint; inferior head—neck of the mandible

- *Muscle Action:* Protrusion of the mandible

- *Injection Localization:* 3 fingerbreadths anterior to the tragus and 1 fingerbreadth inferior to the margin of the zygomatic arch

- *Recommended Number of Injection Sites:* 1

	Botox (units)	Dysport (units)	Xeomin (units)	Myobloc (units)
Suggested Dose	5–30[1,7]	30–100[1,7]	5–30[1,7]	250–1,500*

*Author recommendations.

INJECTION PEARLS AND PITFALLS

If the needle is inserted too superficially or anteriorly, then it will be in the masseter.

11.9 Medial Pterygoid

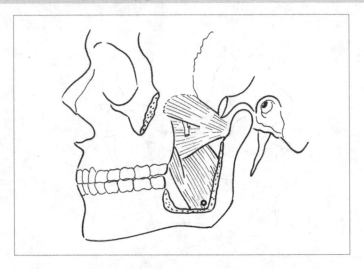

- *Muscle Origin:* Medial surface of the lateral pterygoid plate of the sphenoid bone; maxillary tuberosity

- *Muscle Insertion:* Medial surface of the ramus and angle of the mandible

- *Muscle Action:* Elevation of the mandible, movement of the lower jaw sideways

- *Injection Localization:* Perpendicular to the skin behind the angle of the mandible. Please note: The illustration includes a hollow circle as we want readers to understand that muscle is located behind the jaw and approached inferiorly.

- *Recommended Number of Injection Sites:* 1

	Botox (units)	Dysport (units)	Xeomin (units)	Myobloc (units)
Suggested Dose	5–20[1,7,8]	20–80[1]	5–20[1]	250–1,500*

*Author recommendations.

INJECTION PEARLS AND PITFALLS

This muscle is difficult to inject for a novice injector; consider using a second localization method (such as ultrasound) if injecting for the first time.

11.10 Mentalis

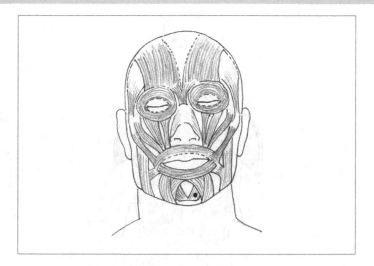

- *Muscle Origin:* Anterior mandible
- *Muscle Insertion:* Chin soft tissue
- *Muscle Action:* Elevating and wrinkling skin of the chin
- *Injection Localization:* 0.5 fingerbreadth lateral from the midline of the chin.
- *Recommended Number of Injection Sites:* 1

	Botox (units)	Dysport (units)	Xeomin (units)	Myobloc (units)
Suggested Dose	1.25–2.5[1]	5–10[1]	1.25–2.5[1]	50–125*

*Author recommendations.

INJECTION PEARLS AND PITFALLS

If the needle is inserted too far laterally, then it will be in the depressor labii. If the needle is inserted too cranially, then it will be in the orbicularis oris.

11.11 Occipitalis

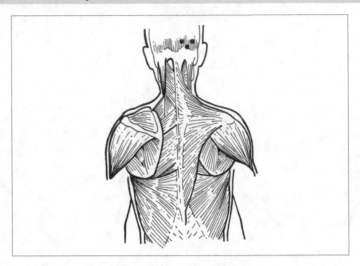

- *Muscle Origin:* Superior nuchal line of the occipital bone and mastoid process of the temporal bone
- *Muscle Insertion:* Galea aponeurosis
- *Muscle Action:* Moves the scalp back
- *Injection Localization:* Site 1: Midpoint of the imaginary line joining the inion and tip of the mastoid process. Site 2: 1 fingerbreadth superior and lateral to Site 1.
- *Recommended Number of Injection Sites:* 1–3

	Botox (units)	Dysport (units)	Xeomin (units)	Myobloc (units)
Suggested Dose	15[†,2]	30–60*	5–15*	250–500*

*Author recommendations.

[†]Denotes FDA-approved dosing.

INJECTION PEARLS AND PITFALLS

If the needle is inserted too inferiorly, then it will be in the cervical paraspinal muscles.

References

1. Jost W. *Pictorial Atlas of Botulinum Toxin Injection*. 2nd ed. Quintessence Publishing Co, Ltd; 2012.
2. Allergan. Botox [package insert]. Published July 2020. https://media .allergan.com/actavis/actavis/media/allergan-pdf-documents/product -prescribing/20190620-BOTOX-100-and-200-Units-v3-0USPI1145-v2 -0MG1145.pdf
3. Allergan. Botox [package insert] cosmetic. Published November 2019. https://media.allergan.com/actavis/actavis/media/allergan-pdf -documents/product-prescribing/20190626-BOTOX-Cosmetic-Insert -72715US10-Med-Guide-v2-0MG1145.pdf
4. Ipsen. Dysport [package insert]. Published September 2019. https://www .ipsen.com/websites/Ipsen_Online/wp-content/uploads/sites/9/2020/ 01/09195739/S115_2019_09_25_sBLA_Approval_PMR_Fulfilled_PI_MG_ Sept-2019.pdf
5. Merz. Xeomin [package insert]. Published August 2020. https://dailymed .nlm.nih.gov/dailymed/fda/fdaDrugXsl.cfm?setid=ccdc3aae-6e2d-4cd0 -a51c-8375bfee9458&type=display
6. Tamura BM, Odo MY, Chang B, et al. Treatment of nasal wrinkles with botulinum toxin. *Dermatol Surg*. 2005;31(3):271–275. doi:10.1111/j.1524-4725 .2005.31072
7. Schwartz M, Freund B. Treatment of temporomandibular disorders with botulinum toxin. *Clin J Pain*. 2002;18(suppl 6):S198–S203. doi:10.1097/ 00002508-200211001-00013
8. Walrath J. Cosmetic use of botulinum toxin. *Rev Ophthalmol*. 2012;19(11): 94–99. https://www.reviewofophthalmology.com/article/cosmetic-use-of -botulinum-toxin

CHAPTER 12

Muscles of the Neck

12.1 Sternocleidomastoid

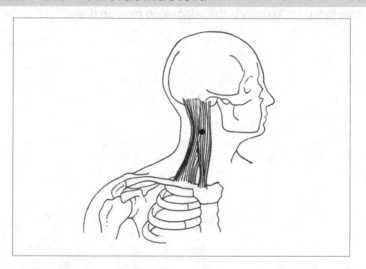

- *Muscle Origin:* Mastoid process
- *Muscle Insertion:* Sternal head—sternum; clavicular head—medial third of the clavicle
- *Muscle Action:* Ipsilateral side bending and contralateral rotation
- *Injection Localization:* With the head turned away, identify the sternal head and measure 4 fingerbreadths cephalad along the muscle from the sternal insertion.
- *Recommended Number of Injection Sites:* 1–3

	Botox® (units)	Dysport® (units)	Xeomin® (units)	Myobloc® (units)
Suggested Dose	15–100[†,1]	50–350[†,2]	20–50[3] (25)[†,4]	1,000–2,500[†,5]

[†]Denotes FDA-approved dosing.

(continued)

INJECTION PEARLS AND PITFALLS

To identify the muscle, have the patient activate the muscle by rotating the head against resistance on the contralateral chin. Inserting the needle too deeply can damage the carotid artery and jugular vein. If the needle is inserted deeply proximal to the clavicle, then there will be a risk of injury to the brachial plexus. There is a risk of dysphagia with bilateral SCM injection. The FDA-approved dose listed for Xeomin is the suggested median dose.

12.2 Scalene Complex

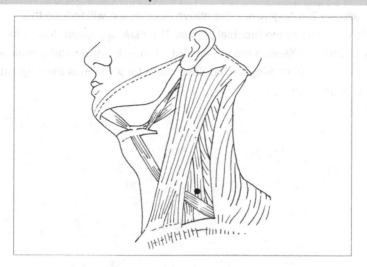

- *Muscle Origin:*

    - Anterior scalene—transverse processes of C3–C6
      Middle scalene—transverse processes of C5–C6
      Posterior Scalene—transverse processes of C4–C6

- *Muscle Insertion:* Anterior and middle scalene—first rib; posterior scalene—second rib

- *Muscle Action:* Unilateral muscles—lateral flexion of the neck and elevation of the first and second rib during inhalation; bilateral muscles—flexion of neck

- *Injection Localization:* 2 fingerbreadths anterior to the edge of the trapezius and 2–4 fingerbreadths above the clavicle

- *Recommended Number of Injection Sites:* 1–3

	Botox (units)	Dysport (units)	Xeomin (units)	Myobloc (units)
Suggested Dose	10–20[†]	50–300[†,2]	10–20*	500–2,000[6,7]
	(15–50)[†,1]		(20)[†,4]	(500–1,000)[†,5]

*Author recommendations.

[†]Denotes FDA-approved dosing.

(continued)

INJECTION PEARLS AND PITFALLS

Injecting 2–4 fingerbreadths above the clavicle will reduce the risk of injury to the brachial plexus. The FDA-approved dosing for Dysport and Xeomin are suggested for anterior and middle scalene muscles. The FDA-approved dose listed for Xeomin is the suggested median dose.

12.3 Longissimus Capitis/Cervicis

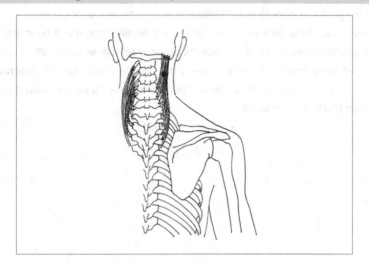

- *Muscle Origin:*
    - Longissimus capitis: Tendons of the longissimus cervicis; articular processes of C4–C8
    - Longissimus cervicis: Transverse processes of T1–T6

- *Muscle Insertion:*
    - Longissimus capitis: Mastoid process of the skull
    - Longissimus cervicis: Transverse processes of C2–C6

- *Muscle Action:* Unilateral activation of the muscle assists with lateral flexion of the cervical spine. Bilateral activation of the muscle assists with extension of the cervical spine.

- *Injection Localization:* 3 fingerbreadths lateral to the midline and 2 fingerbreadths below the lower palpable border of the skull

- *Recommended Number of Injection Sites:* 1

	Botox (units)	Dysport (units)	Xeomin (units)	Myobloc (units)
Suggested Dose	30–50* (30–100)[†,1]	100–200[†,2]	30–50*	1,000–2,000*

*Author recommendations.

[†]Denotes FDA-approved dosing.

(continued)

INJECTION PEARLS AND PITFALLS

Longissimus capitis and longissimus cervicis are contiguous muscles. If the needle is inserted too medially, then it will be in the cervical paraspinals. If the needle is inserted too superficially, then it will be in the levator scapulae. If the needle is inserted too laterally, then it will be in the scalene. There is a risk of anterior head drop with bilateral injections.

12.4 Trapezius

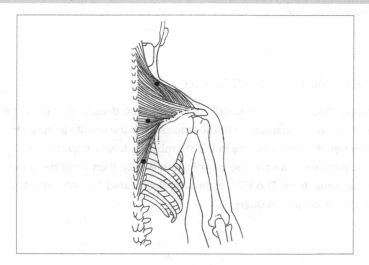

- *Muscle Origin:* External occipital protuberance, ligamentum nuchae, spinous process of C7 and all thoracic vertebrae

- *Muscle Insertion:* Spine of the scapula, lateral third of the clavicle and acromion

- *Muscle Action:* Upper fibers assist with elevation of the scapula. Middle fibers assist with retraction of the scapula. Inferior fibers assist with depression of the scapula and rotation of the glenoid cavity upward.

- *Injection Localization:*
    - Upper fibers: At the curve of the neck and shoulder
    - Middle fibers: 1–2 fingerbreadths medial to the superior angle of the scapula on a horizontal line between the spine of the scapula and the vertebral column
    - Lower: 2 fingerbreadths from the spinous process of the vertebrae at the level of the inferior angle of the scapula

- *Recommended Number of Injection Sites:* 3–6

(continued)

	Botox (units)	Dysport (units)	Xeomin (units)	Myobloc (units)
Suggested Dose	20–100[†,1]	50–300[†,2]	25–100[3,6] (25)[†,4]	1,000–2,500[†,5]

[†]Denotes FDA-approved dosing.

INJECTION PEARLS AND PITFALLS

Upper trapezius: If the needle is inserted too deeply, then it will be in the levator scapulae. Middle trapezius: If the needle is inserted too deeply, then it will be in the rhomboids. Lower trapezius: If the needle is inserted too deeply or inferiorly, then it will be in the latissimus dorsi. The FDA-approved dose listed for Xeomin is the suggested median dose.

12.5 Levator Scapulae

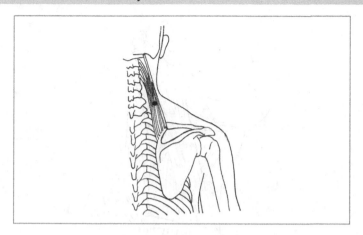

- *Muscle Origin:* Transverse processes of the first four cervical vertebrae
- *Muscle Insertion:* The superior angle and superior part of the medial border of the scapula
- *Muscle Action:* Elevates the scapula
- *Injection Localization:* The anterior edge of the trapezius at the curve of the neck at a point approximately midway between a line joining the transverse process of C1 and the medial angle of the scapula
- *Recommended Number of Injection Sites:* 1–2

	Botox (units)	Dysport (units)	Xeomin (units)	Myobloc (units)
Suggested Dose	20–100[†,1]	50–200[†,2]	20–100[3,6] (25)[†,4]	1,000–2,500[†,5]

[†]Denotes FDA-approved dosing.

INJECTION PEARLS AND PITFALLS

If the needle is inserted too superficially, then it will be in the trapezius. If the needle is inserted too deeply, then it will be in the thoracic paraspinal muscles. There is a risk of anterior head drop with bilateral injections. The FDA-approved dose listed for Xeomin is the suggested median dose.

12.6 Splenius Capitis

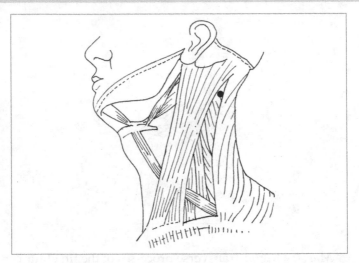

- *Muscle Origin:* Ligamentum nuchae, spinous processes of C7 and T1–T3 or T4

- *Muscle Insertion:* Mastoid process and occipital bone of the skull

- *Muscle Action:* Unilateral activation results in ipsilateral rotation; bilateral activation assists with extension of the head.

- *Injection Localization:* In the upper part of the posterior triangle of the neck, posterior to the sternocleidomastoid and anterior to the trapezius

- *Recommended Number of Injection Sites:* 1

	Botox (units)	Dysport (units)	Xeomin (units)	Myobloc (units)
Suggested Dose	15–100[†,1]	100–350* (75–450)[†,2]	40–100[6,7] (48)[†,4]	1,000–2,500[†,5]

*Author recommendations.

[†]Denotes FDA-approved dosing.

(continued)

INJECTION PEARLS AND PITFALLS

There is a risk of anterior head drop with bilateral injections. The FDA-approved dose listed for Xeomin is the suggested median dose. Xeomin has approval for injection of the splenius capitis and semispinalis capitis combined.

12.7 Splenius Cervicis

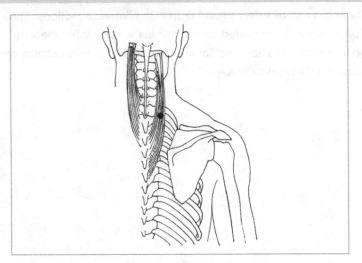

- *Muscle Origin:* Spinous processes of T3–T6
- *Muscle Insertion:* Transverse processes of C2–C4
- *Muscle Action:* Unilateral activation results in ipsilateral rotation of the neck; bilateral activation results in extension of the neck
- *Injection Localization:* 1 fingerbreadth lateral to the T1 spinous process, will pass through the trapezius
- *Recommended Number of Injection Sites:* 1

	Botox (units)	Dysport (units)	Xeomin (units)	Myobloc (units)
Suggested Dose	10–50* (20–60)[†,1]	30–100*	10–50*	1,000–2,500*

*Author recommendations.

[†]Denotes FDA-approved dosing.

INJECTION PEARLS AND PITFALLS

There is a risk of anterior head drop with bilateral injections. This muscle has close proximity to the trapezius, rhomboid minor, splenius capitis, and serratus posterior superior.

12.8 Semispinalis Capitis

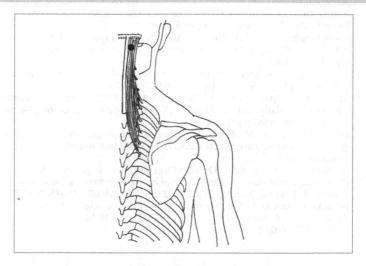

- *Muscle Origin:* Transverse processes of T1–T6/7 and articular processes of C6–C8

- *Muscle Insertion:* Occipital bone

- *Muscle Action:* Extension of head

- *Injection Localization:* 2 fingerbreadths below the occipital protuberance and 2 fingerbreadths away from midline

- *Recommended Number of Injection Sites:* 1

	Botox (units)	Dysport (units)	Xeomin (units)	Mybloc (units)
Suggested Dose	30–100[†,1]	50–250[†,2]	20–100[6] (48)[†,4]	1,000–2,500[†,5]

[†]Denotes FDA-approved dosing.

INJECTION PEARLS AND PITFALLS

There is a risk of anterior head drop with bilateral injection. The FDA-approved dose listed for Xeomin is the suggested median dose. Xeomin has approval for injection of the splenius capitis and semispinalis capitis combined.

References

1. Allergan, ed. *Injection workbook for movement disorders*. Revised May 2018. https://www.botoxmedical.com/Common/Assets/Movement%20 Disorders%20Injection%20Workbook.PDF
2. Ipsen Biopharmaceuticals Inc, ed. Patient injection record: adult cervical dystonia. 2019. https://www.dysporthcp.com/cervical-dystonia/injection-dosing/
3. Tater P, Pandey S. Botulinum toxin in movement disorders. *Neurol India*. 2018;66(suppl):S79–S89. doi:10.4103/0028-3886.226441
4. Merz. Xeomin [package insert]. Published August 2020. https://dailymed.nlm.nih.gov/dailymed/fda/fdaDrugXsl.cfm?setid=ccdc3aae-6e2d-4cd0-a51c-8375bfee9458&type=display
5. US WorldMeds, ed. *Myobloc rimabotulinumtoxinB injection training resource guide*. 2019. https://myoblochcp.com/Cervical-Dystonia/dosing-and-administration
6. Albanese A, Abbruzzese G, Dressler D, et al. Practical guidance for CD management involving treatment of botulinum toxin: a consensus statement. *J Neurol*. 2015;262(10):2201–2213. doi:10.1007/s00415-015-7703-x
7. Benecke R, Dressler D. Botulinum toxin treatment of axial and cervical dystonia. *Disabil Rehabil*. 2007;29(23):1769–1777. doi:10.1080/01421590701568262

CHAPTER 13

Muscles of the Trunk

13.1 Rectus Abdominis

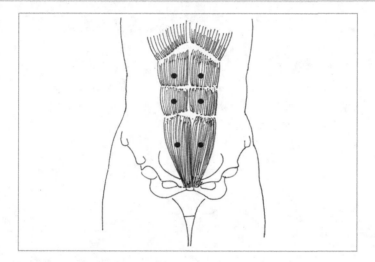

- *Muscle Origin:* Pubic crest and ligaments of the pubic symphysis

- *Muscle Insertion:* Xiphoid process 5–7

- *Muscle Action:* Trunk flexion

- *Injection Localization:* Divide the muscle into three portions: upper, middle, and lower. Insert the needle 2 fingerbreadths lateral to the abdominal midline in each portion. Insert the needle until EMG activity is obtained.

- *Recommended Number of Injection Sites:* 3–6

	Botox® (units)	Dysport® (units)	Xeomin® (units)	Myobloc® (units)
Suggested Dose (each side)	25–100*	40–200[1]	25–100*	1,000–2,500*

*Author recommendations.

(continued)

INJECTION PEARLS AND PITFALLS

If the needle is inserted too deeply, then it will penetrate the peritoneum.

13.2 Internal Oblique

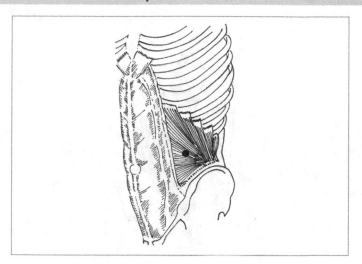

- *Muscle Origin:* Iliopsoas fascia and lateral half of the inguinal ligament, anterior part of the iliac crest, thoracolumbar fascia
- *Muscle Insertion:* Aponeurosis into the linea alba, lower ribs
- *Muscle Action:* Compression of the abdominal cavity, flexion and rotation of the trunk
- *Injection Localization:* Midclavicular line in between the iliac crest and the inferior border of the rib cage
- *Recommended Number of Injection Sites:* 1–4

	Botox (units)	Dysport (units)	Xeomin (units)	Myobloc (units)
Suggested Dose	25–50*	50–150*	25–50*	500–1,500*

*Author recommendations.

INJECTION PEARLS AND PITFALLS

If the needle is inserted too deeply, then it will be in the transversus abdominis or it will penetrate the peritoneum. If the needle is inserted too superficially, then it will be in the external oblique.

13.3 External Oblique

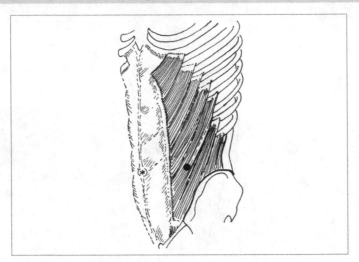

- *Muscle Origin:* Lower six ribs
- *Muscle Insertion:* Anterior part of the iliac crest, pubis, aponeurosis into the linea alba and lower ribs
- *Muscle Action:* Compression of the abdominal cavity; flexion and rotation of the trunk
- *Injection Localization:* Midclavicular line in between the iliac crest and the inferior border of the rib cage. Insert the needle until EMG activity is obtained.
- *Recommended Number of Injection Sites:* 1–4

	Botox (units)	Dysport (units)	Xeomin (units)	Myobloc (units)
Suggested Dose	25–50*	50–150*	25–50*	500–1,500*

*Author recommendations.

INJECTION PEARLS AND PITFALLS

If the needle is inserted too deeply, then it will be in the internal oblique or transverse abdominis and may penetrate the peritoneum.

13.4 Transversus Abdominis

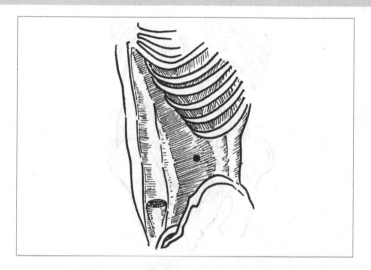

- *Muscle Origin:* Thoracolumbar fascia, lateral part of the inguinal ligament, tips of the lower six ribs and anterior part of the iliac crest

- *Muscle Insertion:* Aponeurosis into the linea alba

- *Muscle Action:* Compression of the abdominal cavity

- *Injection Localization:* Midclavicular line in between the iliac crest and the inferior border of the rib cage

- *Recommended Number of Injection Sites:* 1–4

	Botox (units)	Dysport (units)	Xeomin (units)	Myobloc (units)
Suggested Dose	25–50*	50–150*	25–50*	500–1,500*

*Author recommendations.

INJECTION PEARLS AND PITFALLS

If the needle is inserted too deeply, then it will penetrate the peritoneum. If the needle is inserted too superficially, then it will be in the external or internal oblique.

13.5 Quadratus Lumborum

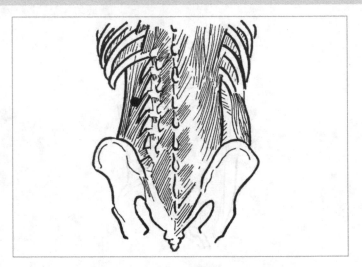

- *Muscle Origin:* Medial part of the iliac crest
- *Muscle Insertion:* Rib 12, lower lumbar vertebrae
- *Muscle Action:* Lateral flexion of the trunk
- *Injection Localization:* 3 fingerbreadths lateral to the spinous processes of the second lumbar vertebrae with the patient in the sphinx position
- *Recommended Number of Injection Sites:* 1–3

	Botox (units)	Dysport (units)	Xeomin (units)	Myobloc (units)
Suggested Dose	50–100*	150–300*	50–100*	2,000–3,000*

*Author recommendations.

INJECTION PEARLS AND PITFALLS

If the needle is inserted too medially, then it will be in the lumbar paraspinal muscles. If the needle is inserted too deeply, then it will be in the psoas muscle or retroperitoneal space.

Reference

1. Jost W. *Pictorial Atlas of Botulinum Toxin Injection*. 2nd ed. Quintessence Publishing Co, Ltd; 2012.

PART V

Other Clinical Applications

CHAPTER 14

Cervical Dystonia

Background

Cervical dystonia (CD) is the most common form of focal dystonia, with a reported prevalence of up to 5 per 100,000 individuals.[1] CD is a heterogeneous disorder characterized by involuntary muscle contractions leading to various abnormal turning or twisting postures of the head, neck, and shoulders. The most commonly encountered posture in clinical practice is torticollis (rotational posture), followed by laterocollis (side tilt), anterocollis (flexion), and retrocollis (extension). Other postures that may be assumed include sagittal shifts or shoulder elevation. Individual postures may occur in isolation, or in a complex presentation of two or more abnormal postures. Torticollis is sometimes accompanied by tremor-like movements that are accentuated by voluntary head turning. Oral therapies such as anticholinergics, benzodiazepines, and muscle relaxants have been used for CD with limited therapeutic benefits and numerous limiting side effects.

Numerous scales have been developed for the evaluation of CD, with various advantages and drawbacks. The Toronto Western Spasmodic Torticollis Rating Scale (TWSTRS) is frequently used in clinical trials and includes three parts: the severity subscale (based on physical findings), the disability subscale, and the pain subscale. Despite its frequent use in clinical trials, the TWSTRS lacks a dystonic tremor component and its complexity limits its use in clinical practice. The Tsui score is another tool frequently employed in clinical trials, and is more streamlined than the TWSTRS scale. The Tsui scale evaluates the rotation, tilt, sagittal movement, head tremor, and shoulder elevation associated with CD, but does not include a rating for shift nor does it evaluate disability or pain. Neither of these scales have been tested rigorously enough to be used to track responsiveness to therapeutic intervention.[2] The Burke-Fahn-Marsden Dystonia Scale and Unified Dystonia Rating Scale are other commonly used dystonia rating scales that have subsections for cervical dystonia but lack the precision to evaluate CD-specific features.[3]

All four commercially available botulinum toxins—
Onabotulinumtoxin A, Abobotulinumtoxin A, Incobotulinumtoxin A, and Rimabotulinumtoxin B—are FDA-approved for
treatment of cervical dystonia in the United States.

Injection Technique and Dosing

Cervical dystonia is a heterogeneous condition that can be com-
prised of various combinations of abnormal postures or positions
(Figures 14.1–14.4); thus, muscle selection must be individualized based on each patient's specific presentation and associated
symptoms such as tremor or pain. For each abnormal posture
in CD, there is a set of primary muscles involved that should be
targeted in all cases (Table 14.1). There is also a set of secondary muscles that may be incorporated in the treatment regimen
if needed due to sub-optimal response. For postures involving
lateral deviation such as torticollis, laterocollis, or lateral shifts,
muscles are injected either ipsilaterally (on the side of deviation)
or contralaterally (opposite the side of deviation). Conversely,
with postures involving deviations in the sagittal plane such as
anterocollis, retrocollis, or sagittal shifts, bilateral neck muscles
are injected symmetrically. For example, in right torticollis, in

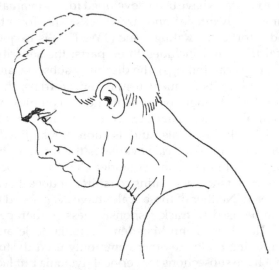

Figure 14.1 Different presentations of cervical dystonia—
anterocollis.

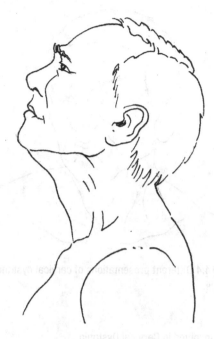

Figure 14.2 Different presentations of
cervical dystonia—retrocollis.

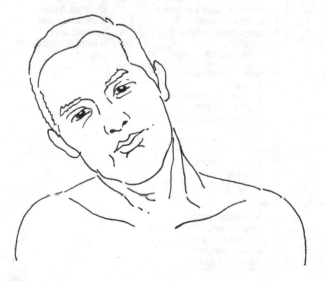

Figure 14.3 Different presentations of cervical dystonia—
laterocollis.

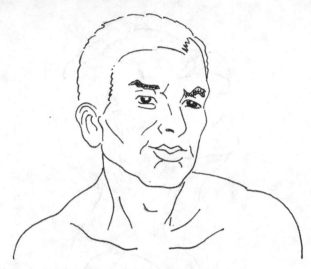

Figure 14.4 Different presentations of cervical dystonia—torticollis.

Table 14.1 Muscles Involved in Cervical Dystonia

Posture	Muscles	
	Ipsilateral	Contralateral
Torticollis	■ Splenius capitis and cervicis ■ Levator scapulae ■ Longissimus capitis and cervicis* ■ Obliquus capitis inferior*	■ Sternocleidomastoid ■ Scalenus complex* ■ Trapezius (upper)* ■ Semispinalis capitis and cervicis*
Laterocollis	■ Sternocleidomastoid ■ Trapezius ■ Splenius capitis and cervicis ■ Scalenus complex ■ Longissimus capitis and cervicis*	
Anterocollis	Bilateral: ■ Sternocleidomastoid ■ Scalenus complex ■ Longus colli*	
Retrocollis	Bilateral: ■ Semispinalis capitis ■ Longissimus capitis and cervicis ■ Splenius capitis and cervicis ■ Levator scapulae* ■ Trapezius (upper)*	

(continued)

Table 14.1 Muscles Involved in Cervical Dystonia (*continued*)

Posture	Muscles	
	Ipsilateral	Contralateral
Shoulder Elevation	■ Trapezius ■ Levator scapulae*	
Lateral Shift	■ Scalenus complex ■ Levator scapulae	■ Sternocleidomastoid ■ Splenius capitis
Sagittal Shift	Bilateral: ■ Sternocleidomastoid	

*Secondary muscle to target if needed.
Sources: Data from Benecke R, Frei K, Comella C. Treatment of cervical dystonia. In: Truong D, Dressler D, Hallett M, eds. *Manual of Botulinum Toxin Therapy.* Cambridge University Press; 2009:29–42; Stacy MA. *Handbook of Dystonia.* CRC Press; 2012.

which the head is turned to the right, you would inject the right splenius capitis ipsilaterally and the left sternocleidomastoid contralaterally. In right laterocollis in which the head tilts to the right, all targeted muscles will be located ipsilaterally on the right.

Please refer to Chapter 12 for anatomic localization of primary muscles. Anatomic localization for longus coli and obliquus capitis inferior, which are secondary muscles for CD, is not recommended. Ultrasonography (US) or fluoroscopic guidance should be used for localization, which is outside the scope of this book.

Numerous guidance methods have been utilized to augment the traditional approach of targeting botulinum neurotoxin injections based on anatomical landmarks, in an effort to optimize botulinum toxin injections for cervical dystonia. These methods include polymyographic electromyography (pEMG), electrical stimulation (e-stim), and US, among others. pEMG is among the most commonly used guidance methods, with robust evidence to support its utility in improving patient outcomes and reducing the incidence of adverse effects.[5] Electrical stimulation of the selected muscle to improve targeting accuracy is another method, though it is more commonly used in limb spasticity.[6] Use of ultrasonographic guidance has gained some ground in recent years, with some evidence to suggest reduced incidence of dysphagia with botulinum neurotoxin injections for CD,[7] though overall expert opinion remains divided on the issue.[5,8] The addition of fluoroscopy or the use of a combination of guidance methods have been used for more challenging presentations to treat muscles such as longus coli.

Complications

The cervical region is fraught with critical structures that must be avoided. In the anterior region, care should be taken to avoid injection deep to the sternocleidomastoid, which contains the pharynx and esophagus, whereby leakage of toxin onto these structures can cause dysphagia and voice changes. Posterior to the sternocleidomastoid, one must take care to avoid the brachial plexus, which passes deep to the scalenus anterior, as well as the inferior belly of the omohyoid, which is just above and deep to the clavicle. If erroneously injected, this can lead to dysphagia.[4]

Clinical Pearls and Pitfalls

- Treatment failure at the onset of therapy (primary non-response) may be attributed to numerous factors such as misdiagnosis, improper injection technique, or improper toxin storage or handling.[9] An important consideration is incomplete muscle selection, particularly in certain complex dystonia postures whereby deeper muscles are implicated in neck deviation, such as the involvement of the longus colli muscles in anterocollis.[10]

- Failure of treatment later in the course of therapy (secondary non-response) can again be attributed to improper injection, toxin handling, or storage; however, an important consideration is development of neutralizing antibodies. The clinical relevance of these antibodies remains under intense debate,[9,11] though greater dosing frequency, use of booster injections, and greater total number of injections has been associated with increased risk of antibodies.[12]

- Current manufacturer guidelines suggest a follow-up period of no less than every 12 weeks,[13-16] though studies have shown that due to a variable response duration in patients,[17] an individualized dosing schedule may be preferable to a fixed 12-week interval schedule.

References

1. Steeves TD, Day L, Dykeman J, et al. The prevalence of primary dystonia: a systematic review and meta-analysis. *Mov Disord.* 2012;27(14):1789–1796. doi:10.1002/mds.25244
2. Jost WH, Hefter H, Stenner A, Reichel G. Rating scales for cervical dystonia: a critical evaluation of tools for outcome assessment of botulinum toxin therapy. *J Neural Transm (Vienna).* 2013;120(3):487–496. doi:10.1007/s00702-012-0887-7
3. Albanese A, Sorbo FD, Comella C, et al. Dystonia rating scales: critique and recommendations. *Mov Disord.* 2013;28(7):874–883. doi:10.1002/mds.25579
4. Stacy MA. *Handbook of Dystonia.* CRC Press; 2012.
5. Contarino MF, Van Den Dool J, Balash Y, et al. Clinical practice: evidence -based recommendations for the treatment of cervical dystonia with botulinum toxin. *Front Neurol.* 2017;8. doi:10.3389/fneur.2017.00035
6. Grigoriu A-I, Dinomais M, Rémy-Néris O, Borchard S. Impact of injection-guiding techniques on the effectiveness of botulinum toxin for the treatment of focal spasticity and dystonia: a systematic review. *Arch Phys Med Rehabil.* 2015;96(11):2067. doi:10.1016/j.apmr.2015.05.002
7. Hong JS, Sathe GG, Niyonkuru C, Munin MC. Elimination of dysphagia using ultrasound guidance for botulinum toxin injections in cervical dystonia. *Muscle Nerve.* 2012;46(4):535–539. doi:10.1002/mus.23409
8. Schramm A, Bäumer T, Fietzek U, et al. Relevance of sonography for botulinum toxin treatment of cervical dystonia: an expert statement. *J Neural Transm.* 2015;122(10):1457–1463. doi:10.1007/s00702-014-1356-2
9. Benecke R. Clinical relevance of botulinum toxin immunogenicity. *BioDrugs.* 2012;26(2):e1–e9. doi:10.2165/11599840-000000000-00000
10. Bhidayasiri R. Treatment of complex cervical dystonia with botulinum toxin: involvement of deep-cervical muscles may contribute to suboptimal responses. *Parkinsonism Relat Disord.* 2011;17(suppl 1):S20–S24. doi:10.1016/j.parkreldis.2011.06.015
11. Bledsoe IO, Comella CL. Botulinum toxin treatment of cervical dystonia. *Semin Neurol.* 2016;36(01):047–053. doi:10.1055/s-0035-1571210
12. Greene P, Fahn S, Diamond B. Development of resistance to botulinum toxin type A in patients with torticollis. *Mov Disord.* 1994;9(2):213–217. doi:10.1002/mds.870090216
13. Allergan. Botox [package insert]. Published July 2020. https://media.allergan.com/actavis/actavis/media/allergan-pdf-documents/product-prescribing/20190620-BOTOX-100-and-200-Units-v3-0USPI1145-v2-0MG1145.pdf
14. Ipsen. Dysport [package insert]. Published September 2019. https://www.ipsen.com/websites/Ipsen_Online/wp-content/uploads/sites/9/2020/01/09195739/S115_2019_09_25_sBLA_Approval_PMR_Fulfilled_PI_MG_Sept-2019.pdf
15. Merz. Xeomin [package insert]. Published August 2020. https://dailymed.nlm.nih.gov/dailymed/fda/fdaDrugXsl.cfm?setid=ccdc3aae-6e2d-4cd0-a51c-8375bfee9458&type=display
16. WorldMeds U. Myobloc [package insert]. Published August 2019. https://myobloc.com/files/MYOBLOC_PI.pdf
17. Misra VP, Ehler E, Zakine B, et al. Factors influencing response to botulinum toxin type A in patients with idiopathic cervical dystonia: results from an international observational study. *BMJ Open.* 2012;2(3):e000881. doi:10.1136/bmjopen-2012-000881.

CHAPTER 15

Chronic Migraine

Background

The International Classification of Headache Disorders is currently the most commonly used paradigm to classify headaches.[1] Migraine-type headaches are one of the most common disabling primary headache disorders; according to the Global Burden of Disease Study, migraines were ranked as the third most prevalent disorder in the world.[2] Chronic migraine (CM) is defined as a headache occurring on 15 or more days per month for more than 3 months with features of migraine on 8 or more days per month.[1] Treatment of CM involves the use of prophylactic treatment.

Onabotulinumtoxin A (OBTA) was approved by the FDA for prophylactic treatment of chronic migraine in 2010. The Phase III Research Evaluating Migraine Prophylaxis Therapy (PREEMPT)-1 and -2 trials have demonstrated that OBTA is a safe, effective, and well-tolerated prophylactic treatment of CM.[3,4] The REal-life use of botulinum toxin for the symptomatic treatment of adults with chronic migraine, measuring healthcare resource utilization, and Patient-reported OutcomeS observed in practice (REPOSE) study also showed that there was a sustained reduction in headache frequency and significant improvement in quality of life measures.[5] OBTA is thought to inhibit nociceptive mediator release from afferent neurons, thereby attenuating peripheral pain signaling to the brain.[6]

There are two patient-report questionnaires that are commonly used when evaluating patients with migraines. The Headache Impact Test 6 (HIT-6) is a 6-item questionnaire that utilizes a Likert scale to assess symptom frequency ranging from "Never" to "Always."[7] Scores range from 36 to 78 with a higher number suggesting higher impact on quality of life. The Migraine Disability Assessment Scale (MIDAS) is a 5-item questionnaire with two additional items. Scores start from 0 and a score above 21 denotes severe disability.[8] HIT-6 is influenced by the intensity and severity of migraines while the MIDAS is influenced by headache frequency.[9] Serial scores can be used to monitor treatment response.

Injection Technique and Dosing

The three most common injection patterns for migraine are a fixed-site approach, "follow the pain" approach, and combination approach.[10] Table 15.1 shows the muscles and dosing for chronic migraine injections for the fixed-site and "follow the pain" approaches. In the fixed-site approach, there are 31 total sites that are injected with 5 units each of OBTA, amounting to a total of 155 units per injection session based on the PREEMPT trial (Figures 15.1–15.3). In the "follow the pain" approach, 2.5 to 5 units are injected at each site with a total maximum dose per session of 195 units. Using this approach, areas of pain and palpable muscle tenderness are clinically identified and injected with 2.5 to 5 units each. Common sites include the frontalis, temporalis, occipitalis, trapezius, splenius capitis, masseter, sternocleidomastoid, or cervical paraspinal muscles.[10,11] The seven specific muscle groups in the fixed-site approach align with the peripheral nerve distributions of the trigeminal, occipital, and cervical sensory nerves.[6] In the combination approach the standard 31 fixed sites are injected and then remaining toxin can be injected into other tender areas.

Table 15.1 Muscles and Dosing for Chronic Migraine Injections

Muscle	Fixed-Site Approach 5 (units/site) Total: 155 units OBTA	"Follow the Pain" Approach 2.5–5 (units/site) Total: Maximum 195 units OBTA
Procerus	1 site (midline)	1 site (midline)
Corrugator	2 sites (1 per side)	2 sites (1 per side)
Frontalis	4 sites (2 per side)	2–4 sites (1–2 per side)
Temporalis	8 sites (4 per side)	8–10 sites (4–5 per side)
Occipitalis	6 sites (3 per side)	6–8 sites (3–4 per side)
Cervical Paraspinals	4 sites (2 per side)	2–6 sites (1–3 per side)
Trapezius	6 sites (3 per side)	2–8 sites (1–4 per side)
Splenius Capitis	–	2–4 sites (1–2 per side)
Masseter	–	2 sites (1 per side)
Sternocleidomastoid	–	2–4 sites (1–2 per side)

OBTA, onabotulinumtoxin A.

Source: Data from Blumenfeld AM, Binder W, Silberstein SD, Blitzer A. Procedures for administering botulinum toxin type A for migraine and tension-type headache. *Headache.* 2003;43(8):884–891. doi:10.1046/j.1526-4610.2003.03167.x

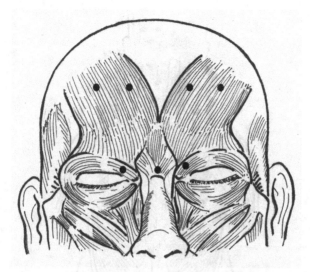

Figure 15.1 Phase III Research Evaluating Migraine Prophylaxis Therapy protocol
migraine injection localization.

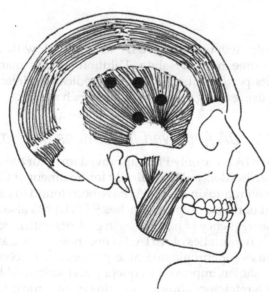

Figure 15.2 Phase III Research Evaluating Migraine Prophylaxis Therapy protocol
migraine injection localization.

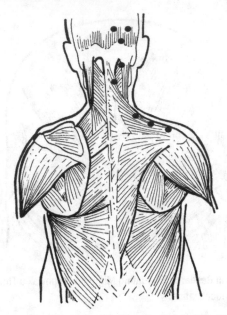

Figure 15.3 Phase III Research Evaluating Migraine Prophylaxis Therapy protocol migraine injection localization.

Commonly 100 units of OBTA are diluted with 2 mL of preservative-free normal saline. Dilution in this manner will yield 5 units per 0.1 mL of prepared medication. Injections are performed using a 30 gauge, 1 inch, or ½ inch needle.

Other Non-FDA Approved Indications and Toxins

Currently, OBTA is the only FDA-approved toxin for the treatment of headache disorders and specifically for treatment of CM. OBTA and Abobotulinumtoxin A (ABTA) have been found to be effective in treatment of tension-type headaches.[12] OBTA has also shown to decrease the frequency of headaches in patients with chronic daily headaches.[13] Two studies of ABTA did not show statistically significant outcomes for chronic migraine prevention. Incobotulinumtoxin A has shown improved frequency and sustained benefit in patients with refractory chronic migraine in one study.[14] Rimabotulinumtoxin B has shown success in patients with inward directed headache (imploding) and those with auras in one study.[15]

Complications

The most common adverse effects from the REPOSE and PRE-EMPT trials include ptosis, neck pain, and musculoskeletal stiffness or weakness.[5,16] Less common and theoretical side effects include injection site pain, bruising, bleeding, generalized weakness, anaphylaxis, allergic reactions, and death.

Clinical Pearls and Pitfalls

- The needle should be inserted at 90-degree for corrugator and procerus and at a 45-degree angle when infecting frontalis. Inserting the needle too deeply may result in hitting the periosteum, which can cause headache.

- For procerus and corrugator, if injections are performed too superiorly, then frontalis may be weakened unintentionally causing brow ptosis.

- The cervical paraspinal muscle group consists of the trapezius, splenius capitis, splenius cervicis, and semispinalis capitis and has been discussed separately in prior chapters. In the PREEMPT trial, 2 sites are injected on each side and injections are kept in the superficial plane and inside the hairline to prevent neck weakness and pain.[6]

- The functional anatomy, injection technique, and pitfalls are discussed in the article by Blumenfeld, 2017.[6]

References

1. Headache Classification Committee of the International Headache Society. *The International Classification of Headache Disorders*, 3rd edition. *Cephalalgia.* 2018;38(1):1–211. doi:10.1177/0333102417738202
2. Saylor D, Steiner TJ. The global burden of headache. *Semin Neurol.* 2018;38(2):182–190. doi:10.1055/s-0038-1646946
3. Aurora SK, Dodick DW, Turkel CC, et al. Onabotulinumtoxin A for treatment of chronic migraine: results from the double-blind, randomized, placebo-controlled phase of the PREEMPT 1 trial. *Cephalalgia.* 2010;30(7):793–803. doi:10.1177/0333102410364676

4. Diener HC, Dodick DW, Aurora SK, et al. Onabotulinumtoxin A for treatment of chronic migraine: results from the double-blind, randomized, placebo-controlled phase of the PREEMPT 2 trial. *Cephalalgia*. 2010;30(7):804–814. doi:10.1177/0333102410364677

5. Ahmed F, Gaul C, Garcia-Moncó JC, et al. An open-label prospective study of the real-life use of Onabotulinumtoxin A for the treatment of chronic migraine: the REPOSE study. *J Headache Pain*. 2019;20(1):26. doi:10.1186/s10194-019-0976-1

6. Blumenfeld AM, Silberstein SD, Dodick DW, et al. Insights into the functional anatomy behind the PREEMPT injection paradigm: guidance on achieving optimal outcomes. *Headache*. 2017;57(5):766–777. doi:10.1111/head.13074

7. Kosinski M, Bayliss MS, Bjorner JB, et al. A six-item short-form survey for measuring headache impact: the HIT-6. *Qual Life Res*. 2003;12(8):963–974. doi:10.1023/A:1026119331193

8. Stewart WF, Lipton RB, Dowson AJ, Sawyer J. Development and testing of the Migraine Disability Assessment (MIDAS) questionnaire to assess headache-related disability. *Neurology*. 2001;56(suppl 1):S20–S28. doi:10.1212/WNL.56.suppl_1.S20

9. Sauro KM, Rose MS, Becker WJ, et al. HIT-6 and MIDAS as measures of headache disability in a headache referral population. *Headache*. 2010;50(3):383–395. doi:10.1111/j.1526-4610.2009.01544.x

10. Blumenfeld AM, Binder W, Silberstein SD, Blitzer A. Procedures for administering botulinum toxin type A for migraine and tension-type headache. *Headache*. 2003;43(8):884–891. doi:10.1046/j.1526-4610.2003.03167.x

11. Silberstein SD. The use of botulinum toxin in the management of headache disorders. *Semin Neurol*. 2016;36(1):92–98. doi:10.1055/s-0036-1571443

12. Wieckiewicz M, Grychowska N, Zietek M, et al. Evidence to use botulinum toxin injections in tension-type headache management: a systematic review. *Toxins (Basel)*. 2017;9(11). doi:10.3390/toxins9110370

13. Mathew NT, Frishberg BM, Gawel M, et al. Botulinum toxin type A (BOTOX) for the prophylactic treatment of chronic daily headache: a randomized, double-blind, placebo-controlled trial. *Headache*. 2005;45(4):293–307. doi:10.1111/j.1526-4610.2005.05066.x

14. Ion I, Renard D, Le Floch A, et al. Monocentric prospective study into the sustained effect of Incobotulinumtoxin A (XEOMIN®) botulinum toxin in chronic refractory migraine. *Toxins (Basel)*. 2018;10(6). doi:10.3390/toxins10060221

15. Grogan PM, Alvarez MV, Jones L. Headache direction and aura predict migraine responsiveness to Rimabotulinumtoxin B. *Headache*. 2013;53(1):126–136. doi:10.1111/j.1526-4610.2012.02288.x

16. Dodick DW, Turkel CC, DeGryse RE, et al. Onabotulinumtoxin A for treatment of chronic migraine: pooled results from the double-blind, randomized, placebo-controlled phases of the PREEMPT clinical program. *Headache*. 2010;50(6):921–936. doi:10.1111/j.1526-4610.2010.01678.x

CHAPTER 16

Blepharospasm

Background

Blepharospasm is a focal dystonia characterized by involuntary, repetitive, and synchronized contractions of the orbicularis oculi, as well as some surrounding muscles, which lead to forceful eyelid closure of both eyes. This is a physically and socially debilitating condition that interferes with visual performance, quality of life, and activities of daily living. In severe cases, this can cause functional blindness. While the etiology is not well understood, previous studies suggest a central origin related to a dysfunction of the basal ganglia, thalamus, and brainstem.[1] Botulinum toxin injections are considered the treatment of choice for blepharospasm.[2] The therapeutic value is a result of the toxin's ability to cause chemodenervation, resulting in a local paralytic effect of the injected muscle. There are several scales that exist to measure the severity of blepharospasm. The most widely used scale is the Jankovic Rating Scale, which measures the frequency and intensity of the blepharospasms.[3] Other scales include the Burke-Fahn-Marsden Dystonia Scale, the Unified Dystonia Rating Scale, and the Global Dystonia Severity Rating Scale, which are not specific to blepharospasm but instead measure severity of dystonia in all body parts.[4]

Onabotulinumtoxin A (Botox®) and Incobotulinumtoxin A (Xeomin®) are the only two formulations that currently have FDA approval for the treatment of blepharospasm.

Injection Technique and Dosing

The orbicularis oculi muscle consists of two components: the orbital and palpebral portions. Both parts narrow the palpebral fissure and the palpebral part is additionally responsible for the blinking reflex.

Injections are placed in medial and lateral areas of the upper eyelid and lateral areas in the lower eyelid. Additional injections can be placed in the nearby corrugator and procerus muscles if they are also involved (Figure 16.1).

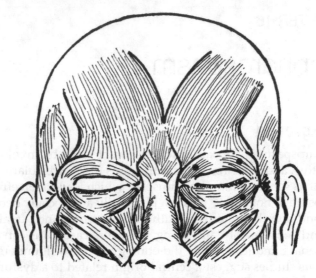

Figure 16.1 Injection points for treatment of blepharospasm.

Typically, anatomical localization is sufficient for injection of botulinum toxin in treatment of blepharospasm. Electromyography, ultrasound, or additional guidance methods are not used for injection in blepharospasm.

Recommended dosing for each injection site is listed in Table 16.1.

Complications

Botulinum toxin B (Myobloc®) is not typically used for the treatment of blepharospasm as side effects of pain on injection and dry eyes occur at a higher frequency than Botulinum toxin A,

Table 16.1 Muscles, Toxins, and Injection Doses for Blepharospasm

Muscle Name	Botox (units/site)	Xeomin (units/site)	Dysport® (units/site)	Myobloc (units/site)
Orbicularis oculi: medial upper lid	1.25–5[5]	1.25–5[5]	5–20[5]	—
Orbicularis oculi: lateral upper lid	1.25–5[5]	1.25–5[5]	5–20[5]	—
Orbicularis oculi: lateral epicanthus	5–10*	5–10*	5–20*	—
Orbicularis oculi: lateral lower lid	2.5–5[5]	2.5–5[5]	5–20[5]	—
Corrugator[†]	2.5–5*	2.5–5*	10–20*	—
Procerus[†]	2.5–5*	2.5–5*	10–20*	—

*Author recommendations.

[†]Denotes optional muscles.

suggesting that it spreads more diffusely.[6] Ecchymosis can easily occur in the soft tissue of the eyelids. To limit this risk, make sure to apply immediate gentle pressure with gauze to the injection site.[5]

Clinical Pearls and Pitfalls

- When targeting the orbicularis oculi muscles, the needle should be inserted parallel to the skin surface.

- When targeting corrugator and procerus muscles, injections should be perpendicular to the skin surface.

- Injections too close to the levator palpebrae superioris can cause ptosis.

- Injections of the medial lower lid can spread to the inferior oblique muscle and cause diplopia.

- Injections in the pars lacrimalis can cause disturbance in the flow of lacrimal fluid, leading to dry eyes.

- Injections too close to the lower margin of the lid can cause ectropion.

- Injections into muscles of the lower face (levator labii superioris alaeque nasi) may cause lower facial palsy.

References

1. Vivancos-Matellano F, Rodriguez-Sanz A, Herrero-Infante Y, Mascías-Cadavid J. Efficacy and safety of long-term therapy with type A botulinum toxin in patients with blepharospasm. *Neuroophthalmology*. 2019;43(5): 277–283. doi:10.1080/01658107.2018.1542009

2. Simpson DM, Hallett M, Ashman EJ, et al. Practice guideline update summary: botulinum neurotoxin for the treatment of blepharospasm, cervical dystonia, adult spasticity, and headache: Report of the Guideline Development Subcommittee of the American Academy of Neurology. *Neurology*. 2016;86(19):1818–1826. doi:10.1212/WNL.0000000000002560

3. Jankovic J, Kenney C, Grafe S, et al. Relationship between various clinical outcome assessments in patients with blepharospasm. *Mov Disord*. 2009;24(3):407–413. doi:10.1002/mds.22368

4. Albanese A, Sorbo FD, Comella C, et al. Dystonia rating scales: critique and recommendations. *Mov Disord*. 2013;28(7):874–883. doi:10.1002/mds.25579

5. Jost W, Valerius KP. *Pictorial Atlas of Botulinum Toxin Injection: Dosage, Localization, Application*. Quintessence Publishing Co, Ltd; 2013.

6. Dutton JJ, White JJ, Richard MJ. Myobloc® for the treatment of benign essential blepharospasm in patients refractory to Botox. *Ophthalmic Plast Reconstr Surg*. 2006;22(3):173–177. doi:10.1097/01.iop.0000217382.33972.c4

CHAPTER 17

Hyperhidrosis

Background

Hyperhidrosis, or increased production of sweat, can affect many aspects of a patient's life. Hyperhidrosis may impact daily activities including the ability to maintain skin hygiene, which can lead to infections. Hyperhidrosis can impact quality of life and interpersonal relationships due to embarrassment from excessive sweating during handshakes, visual stains on clothing, and adverse cosmetic appearance.[1]

Hyperhidrosis can be generalized, involving the whole body, or focal, involving one body part, most commonly the face, armpits, palmar surfaces of hands and feet, or the residual limb after amputation. According to surveys, focal hyperhidrosis affects approximately 2% to 3% of the population in the United States, typically people between the ages of 24 to 65. Men and women are affected equally.[1,2]

The pathophysiology of hyperhidrosis is poorly understood. The human body has approximately 3 to 4 million eccrine sweat glands, which are innervated by cholinergic fibers of the autonomic nervous system; these can be impacted by emotional and gustatory stimuli.[1] Focal hyperhidrosis represents a dysfunction of the autonomic nervous system.[1] Botulinum toxin is one of the many treatment options for hyperhidrosis. When injected intradermally, botulinum toxin blocks the release of acetylcholine from the sympathetic nerve fibers that stimulate sweat glands.[2]

Generalized hyperhidrosis is typically associated with other conditions (Box 17.1). Focal hyperhidrosis is usually idiopathic, but may be associated with other conditions (Box 17.2).[1,2]

History and examination are the first steps in diagnosing hyperhidrosis. Laboratory testing and imaging may be indicated to rule out underlying disorders. Sweat testing using a starch-iodine test is used to diagnose primary idiopathic hyperhidrosis and localize areas of activity to guide injection localization.[3]

The Hyperhidrosis Disease Severity Scale is a qualitative measure of the impact of excessive sweating on activities of daily living (Box 17.3).[2] The Hyperhidrosis Disease Severity Scale may

Box 17.1: Causes of generalized hyperhidrosis

- Endocrine: hyperthyroidism, hypopituitarism, diabetes mellitus, menopause, pregnancy, carcinoid syndrome, acromegaly, pheochromocytoma
- Neurologic: Parkinson's disease, spinal cord injury, cerebro-vascular accident
- Malignant disease: myeloproliferative disorders, Hodgkin's disease
- Infection: cardiovascular shock, heart failure
- Respiratory disorders
- Drugs: fluoxetine, venlafaxine, doxepin
- Toxicity: alcoholism

Source: Reproduced with permission from Haider A, Solish N. Focal hyperhidrosis: diagnosis and management. *CMAJ.* 2005;172(1):69–75. doi:10.1503/cmaj.1040708

Box 17.2: Causes of focal hyperhidrosis

- Primary idiopathic hyperhidrosis
- Gustatory sweating (Frey's syndrome)
- Neurologic: neuropathy, spinal cord injury

Source: Reproduced with permission from Haider A, Solish N. Focal hyperhidrosis: diagnosis and management. *CMAJ.* 2005;172(1):69–75. doi:10.1503/cmaj.1040708

Box 17.3: The Hyperhidrosis Disease Severity Scale (HDSS)

Q: How would you rate the severity of your sweating?

1. Sweating is never noticeable and never interferes with daily activities.
2. Sweating is tolerable and sometimes interferes with daily activities.

(continued)

3. Sweating is barely tolerable and frequently interferes with daily activities.

4. Sweating is intolerable and always interferes with daily activities.

Note: Only severity scores of 3 and 4 should be assigned to true hyperhidrosis.

Source: Reproduced with permission from Truong D, Hallett M, Zachary CB, Dressler D, eds. *Manual of Botulinum Toxin Therapy.* 2nd ed. Cambridge University Press; 2014.

be used for initial evaluation and to monitor treatment response.[2,4] The Keller questionnaire is a specific questionnaire for hyperhidrosis that evaluates the social, emotional, work, and daily activities and conditions including symptoms related to palmar hyperhidrosis. It consists of 15 questions that consider the stress level, scoring from 0 (none) to 10 (worst), of possible various situations of everyday life. Scores above 100 are indicative of severe cases, and those above 125 are very serious.[2]

Injection Technique and Dosing

The injection area is marked in a grid pattern with each point 1 to 2 cm apart from the other. As injections can be painful, topical anesthetics, ice packs, or cold spray may be used for patient comfort. Suggested injection patterns are illustrated in the following figures (Figures 17.1–17.5). A 30 gauge, half- or 1-inch needle may be used.

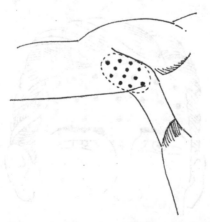

Figure 17.1 Injection points for treatment of axillary hyperhidrosis.

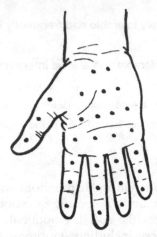

Figure 17.2 Injection points for treatment of palmar hyperhidrosis.

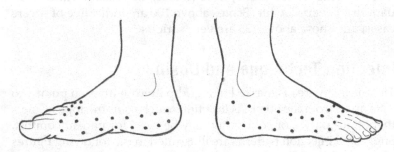

Figure 17.3 Injection points for treatment of plantar hyperhidrosis.

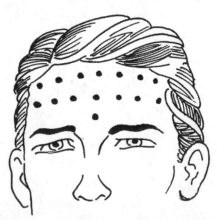

Figure 17.4 Injection points for treatment of frontal illustration.

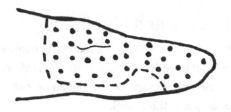

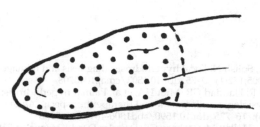

Figure 17.5 Injection points for treatment of residual limb hyperhidrosis.

The toxin should be injected intradermally, holding the needle at a 45° angle to prevent backflow. Suggested dosing is noted in Table 17.1.

Complications

The most common side effects are pain, swelling, and bruising at the injection area.[3]

Table 17.1 Suggested Dosing per Body Area in Units, per Side

Site	Botox®	Dysport®	Xeomin®	Myobloc®
Axilla	50[†,5] 50[3,4,6]	200[3,6]	50[3,6]	2,500*
Palm	100[3,6]	300–400[3,6]	100[3,6]	4,000*
Plantar	100[2,3,6]	300–400[6]	100*	5,000*
Frontal	50–100*	150–200*	50–100*	2,500*
Residual limb	100*	300*	100*	5,000*

†Denotes FDA-approved dosing.

*Author recommendations.

Clinical Pearls and Pitfalls

- It is recommended to have a follow-up evaluation in 2 to 4 weeks post injection using the standard life quality measures. Future treatment plans will be based on patient satisfaction and changes in the HDSS.

- Cost of treatment and limited insurance coverage limits this treatment for common use.

References

1. Haider A, Solish N. Focal hyperhidrosis: diagnosis and management. *CMAJ.* 2005;172(1):69–75. doi:10.1503/cmaj.1040708
2. Romero FR, Haddad GR, Miot HA, et al. Palmar hyperhidrosis: clinical, pathophysiological, diagnostic and therapeutic aspects. *An Bras Dermatol.* 2016;91(6):716–725. doi:10.1590/abd1806-4841.20165358
3. Truong D, Hallett M, Zachary CB, Dressler D, eds. *Manual of Botulinum Toxin Therapy.* 2nd ed. Cambridge University Press; 2014.
4. McConaghy JR, Fosselman D. Hyperhidrosis: management options. *Am Fam Physician.* 2018;97(11):729–734. https://www.aafp.org/afp/2018/0601/p729.html
5. Allergan. Botox [package insert]. Published July 2020. https://media.allergan.com/actavis/actavis/media/allergan-pdf-documents/product-prescribing/20190620-BOTOX-100-and-200-Units-v3-0USPI1145-v2-0MG1145.pdf
6. Jost W. *Pictorial Atlas of Botulinum Toxin Injection.* 2nd ed. Quintessence Publishing Co, Ltd; 2012.

CHAPTER 18

Sialorrhea

Background

Sialorrhea, or drooling, is the involuntary loss of saliva from the mouth.[1] Drooling may be seen in a variety of pathologic conditions including cerebral palsy, acquired brain injury, neurodegenerative disease (such as amyotrophic lateral sclerosis or Parkinson's disease), head and neck carcinomas, and salivary fistulas.[2] Drooling can cause skin maceration, lead to recurrent respiratory infection, and significantly impact community participation and interpersonal relationships for people with disabilities.[1,3] Drooling may be caused by a combination of factors including saliva overproduction, disordered swallowing, and decreased oral saliva management.

On average, adults produce 500 to 1,500 mL of saliva per day.[4] The submandibular gland contributes approximately 70% of total saliva production, the parotid gland contributes 25%, and the sublingual gland contributes about 5%.[3,5] The salivary glands are innervated by parasympathetic nerves and acetylcholine is the transmitter at the neurosecretory junction. Botulinum neurotoxin inhibits acetylcholine transmission from cholinergic nerve endings when delivered intraglandularly, thereby reducing saliva release.[3]

Evaluation of sialorrhea may involve a multidisciplinary team, involving dentists, therapists, and physicians.[2] Measures such as the Drooling Severity and Frequency Scale,[6] Drooling Impact Scale,[7] and Drool Quotient[8] may be used for evaluations initially and for monitoring response to treatment.[9]

Injection Technique and Dosing

The salivary glands can be located using ultrasound imaging or surface anatomical landmarks. Anatomic guidance for injection of the salivary glands is as follows (Figure 18.1)[10]:

- *Parotid Gland:* One fingerbreadth anterior to the midpoint of a line between the tragus and angle of the mandible
- *Submandibular Gland:* One fingerbreadth medial to the midpoint of a line between the inferior edge of the angle of the mandible and the inferior tip of the chin.

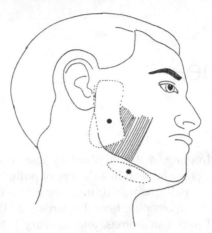

Figure 18.1 Injection points for treatment of sialorrhea.

Table 18.1 Suggested Dosing for Treatment of Sialorrhea

Muscle Name	Botox®	Dysport®	Xeomin®	Myobloc®
Submandibular (units/side)	10–50[2]	15–75[2]	20[†,11]	250[†,10]
Parotid (units/side)	10–50[2]	15–75[2]	30[†,11]	500–1,500[†,10]

[†]Denotes FDA-approved indication.

Typically, one injection is performed in each of the glands (Table 18.1).

Complications

Post-injection complications may include unintended diffusion into muscles of mastication or swallowing. Thickened saliva and dry mouth may lead to difficulties with managing dry food in the oral phase of swallow. Other complications of the injection itself may include intraoral bleeding caused by bleeding at the gland or duct due to injection trauma, or injury to the facial nerve during the course of parotid injections.[2]

Clinical Pearls and Pitfalls

- Injections may be repeated as soon as every 12 weeks, except for Incobotulinumtoxin A in which studies suggest dosing every 16 weeks.[10,11]

References

1. Blasco PA. Surgical management of drooling. *Dev Med Child Neurol.* 1992;34(4):368–369. doi:10.1111/j.1469-8749.1992.tb11444.x
2. Reddihough D, Erasmus CE, Johnson H, et al. Botulinum toxin assessment, intervention and aftercare for paediatric and adult drooling: international consensus statement. *Eur J Neurol.* 2010;17(suppl 2):109–121. doi:10.1111/j.1468-1331.2010.03131.x
3. Tan EK. Botulinum toxin treatment of sialorrhea: comparing different therapeutic preparations. *Eur J Neurol.* 2006;13(suppl 1):60–64. doi:10.1111/j.1468-1331.2006.01447.x
4. Humphrey SP, Williamson RT. A review of saliva: normal composition, flow, and function. *J Prosthet Dent.* 2001;85(2):162–169. doi:10.1067/mpr.2001.113778
5. Jost WH, Bäumer T, Laskawi R, et al. Therapy of sialorrhea with botulinum neurotoxin. *Neurol Ther.* 2019;8(2):273–288. doi:10.1007/s40120-019-00155-6
6. Thomas-Stonell N, Greenberg J. Three treatment approaches and clinical factors in the reduction of drooling. *Dysphagia.* 1988;3(2):73–78. doi:10.1007/BF02412423
7. Reid SM, Johnson HM, Reddihough DS. The drooling impact scale: a measure of the impact of drooling in children with developmental disabilities. *Dev Med Child Neurol.* 2010;52(2):e23–e28. doi:10.1111/j.1469-8749.2009.03519.x
8. Rapp D. Management of drooling. *Dev Med Child Neurol.* 1988;30(1):128–129. doi:10.1111/j.1469-8749.1988.tb04738.x
9. Rashnoo P, Daniel SJ. Drooling quantification: correlation of different techniques. *Int J Pediatr Otorhinolaryngol.* 2015;79(8):1201–1205. doi:10.1016/j.ijporl.2015.05.010
10. WorldMeds US. Myobloc [package insert]. Published August 2019. https://myobloc.com/files/MYOBLOC_PI.pdf
11. Merz. Xeomin [package insert]. Published August 2020. https://dailymed.nlm.nih.gov/dailymed/fda/fdaDrugXsl.cfm?setid=ccdc3aae-6e2d-4cd0-a51c-8375bfee9458&type=display

CHAPTER 19

Chemodenervation of the Lower Urinary Tract

Background

Normal urinary function is an elegant and complex process. Bladder dysfunction arising as a result of a neurological disorder can result in disorders of either bladder storage or emptying. Disorders of storage of urine can often be due to an overactive detrusor or an incompetent urethral sphincter, whereas issues with emptying of urine can be related to an underactive bladder, obstructed urethra, or hyperactive sphincter. The usage of Onabotulinumtoxin A has been described to help with overactive bladder and a hyperactive or dyssynergic external urethral sphincter.

Overactive bladder syndrome is defined by a sensation of urinary urgency with or without urinary urge incontinence.[1] Overactive bladder can be idiopathic or can be neurogenic in origin. Those with neurogenic detrusor overactivity have a presumed neurological cause for their bladder dysfunction, such as spinal cord injury, multiple sclerosis, Parkinson's disease, or cerebral vascular accident.[2] Detrusor external sphincter dyssynergia (DESD) occurs when the sphincter pathologically contracts during an involuntary bladder contraction. This typically occurs in patients with a suprasacral spinal cord lesion (including multiple sclerosis) or injury and can manifest as urinary incontinence, frequency, urgency, retention, or obstructive voiding symptoms.[3]

When attempting to decipher the exact etiology of voiding dysfunction, urodynamics play an important role in distinguishing whether a patient has an issue with storage, emptying, or both. Urodynamics allow the clinician to diagnose detrusor overactivity (DO), detrusor overactivity incontinence (DOI), and detrusor sphincter dyssynergia, as well as a myriad of other storage and emptying disorders.

The use of botulinum toxin in the lower urinary tract was first described in 1987, when it was injected into the external urethral sphincter (EUS) to treat detrusor sphincter dyssynergia.[4] Since that time the use of botulinum toxin in the lower urinary tract

Table 19.1 Indications and Target Muscle

Indication	Target Muscle
Detrusor External Sphincter Dyssynergia (DESD)	External urethral sphincter muscle
Idiopathic and Neurogenic Detrusor Overactivity	Detrusor muscle of the bladder
Bladder Pain Syndrome/Interstitial Cystitis	

system has expanded, and as of 2013, Botox® has been the only botulinum toxin to be FDA-approved to treat both idiopathic and neurogenic detrusor overactivity that is refractory to oral medications. Use of Onabotulinumtoxin A for DESD as well as bladder pain syndrome/interstitial cystitis has been described, though remains off-label. Also, any use of products other than Botox (such as Dysport® noted in Table 19.2) are considered off-label and have not been approved for urological use.

The mechanism of action of botulinum toxin in the bladder is believed to be due to temporary prevention of parasympathetic presynaptic release of acetylcholine, thereby interfering with the efferent nerve stimulation of the detrusor muscle.[5] Additionally, there has been data that botulinum toxin may affect bladder sensation by modulating afferent nerve signaling during bladder filling (Table 19.1).[6]

Injection Technique and Dosing

Bladder Injection

Injections are performed via direct visualization through either a flexible or rigid cystoscope and can be performed under local anesthesia or monitored intravenous sedation. The patient is typically placed in the dorsal lithotomy position, prepped and draped in the standard fashion, and a cystoscope is inserted into the urethra and bladder. The posterior and lateral walls of the bladder are visualized and injected cystoscopically with equally spaced injections approximately 1 to 2 cm apart. During the injection, care is taken to avoid the ureteral orifices located bilaterally. The injection needle is placed submucosally at a depth of 3 to 5 mm.

The original template and FDA approval include 20 injection sites excluding the trigone (Figure 19.1). Recent evidence suggests that injecting fewer sites may result in the same efficacy. There is additional evidence that trigone-including injection techniques may have a superior efficacy with a similar rate of complications (Figure 19.2).[7]

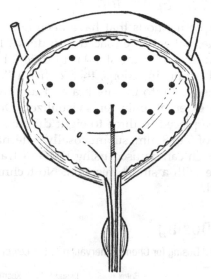

Figure 19.1 Injection points for chemodenervation of lower urinary tract, trigone-sparing.

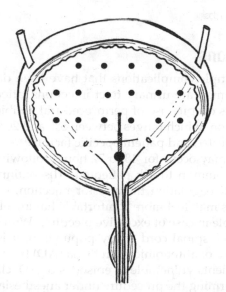

Figure 19.2 Injection points for chemodenervation of lower urinary tract, trigone-including.

External Urethral Sphincter

There are multiple methods that have been described. Regardless of technique, patients are placed into dorsal lithotomy and are prepped and draped in the standard fashion. If the patient is to undergo endoscopic injections, then either a flexible or rigid cystoscope is inserted into the urethra and urethroscopy is performed until the external sphincter is visualized. Once visualized, injections can be placed in three to eight different sites into the EUS at a depth of 3 to 8 mm, submucosally. Alternatively, a transperineal approach can be used using EMG or transrectal ultrasound guidance with a single injection. No technique has been widely accepted.[8]

Suggested Dosing

Table 19.2 Suggested Dosing for Chemodenervation of the Lower Urinary Tract

Indication/Muscle	Botox	Dysport	Xeomin®	Myobloc®
Idiopathic DO/Detrusor Muscle	100 units[†,9]	—	—	—
Neurogenic DO/Detrusor Muscle	200 units[†,10]	750 units[11]	—	—
BPS/IC/Detrusor Muscle	100 units[12]	—	—	—
DESD/External Urethral Sphincter	100 units[13]	—	—	—

[†]Denotes FDA-approved dosing.

Complications

There are multiple complications that have been described; the two most common are urinary tract infections, affecting 20% to 35% of patients despite use of periprocedural antibiotics,[14,15] and urinary retention, which ranges between 5% and 20% depending on the dose injected and patient-specific factors.[14,16]

Hematuria may occur for 48 to 72 hours following the procedure. It is uncommon to ask patients to discontinue their antiplatelet or anticoagulation therapy for injection, but in certain cases clinicians may feel more comfortable having electrocautery readily available in case of excessive bleeding. While performing injections in the spinal cord injury population, it is possible to induce episodes of autonomic dysreflexia (AD) from bladder distention. In patients vulnerable to episodes of AD, clinicians may consider performing the procedure under anesthesia with immediate access to blood pressure-lowering agents.

Clinical Pearls and Pitfalls

- All patients should undergo a urinalysis the day of treatment to ensure that they do not have a urinary tract infection. Injecting in the setting of a urinary tract infection is contra-indicated, and periprocedural prophylaxis is indicated as detailed in the American Urologic Association's best practice statement on antimicrobial prophylaxis.

- If performing this procedure in the office, the patient should receive an intraurethral instillation of 1% to 2% lidocaine, which should be allowed to dwell for at least 20 minutes prior to the procedure.

- Following injection, patients are seen 2 to 4 weeks later to assess symptom improvement and to obtain a post-void residual to ensure patients are adequately emptying.

References

1. Drake MJ. Fundamentals of terminology in lower urinary tract function. *Neurourol Urodyn*. 2018;37(S6):S13–S19. doi:10.1002/nau.23768

2. Gajewski JB, Schurch B, Hamid R, et al. An International Continence Society (ICS) report on the terminology for adult neurogenic lower urinary tract dysfunction (ANLUTD). *Neurourol Urodyn*. 2018;37(3):1152–1161. doi:10.1002/nau.23397

3. Cooley LF, Kielb S. A review of botulinum toxin A for the treatment of neurogenic bladder. *PM R*. 2019;11(2):192–200. doi:10.1016/j.pmrj.2018.07.016

4. Dykstra DD, Sidi AA, Scott AB, et al. Effects of botulinum A toxin on detrusor-sphincter dyssynergia in spinal cord injury patients. *J Urol*. 1988;139(5):919–922. doi:10.1016/S0022-5347(17)42717-0

5. Malde S, Fry C, Schurch B, et al. What is the exact working mechanism of botulinum toxin A and sacral nerve stimulation in the treatment of overactive bladder/detrusor overactivity? ICI-RS 2017. *Neurourol Urodyn*. 2018;37(S4):S108–S116. doi:10.1002/nau.23552

6. Apostolidis A, Dasgupta P, Fowler CJ. Proposed mechanism for the efficacy of injected botulinum toxin in the treatment of human detrusor overactivity. *Eur Urol*. 2006;49(4):644–650. doi:10.1016/j.eururo.2005.12.010

7. Jo JK, Kim KN, Kim DW, et al. The effect of OnabotulinumtoxinA according to site of injection in patients with overactive bladder: a systematic review and meta-analysis. *World J Urol*. 2018;36(2):305–317. doi:10.1007/s00345-017-2121-6

8. Utomo E, Groen J, Blok BF. Surgical management of functional bladder outlet obstruction in adults with neurogenic bladder dysfunction. *Cochrane Database Syst Rev*. 2014;(5):CD004927. doi:10.1002/14651858.CD004927.pub4

9.   Nambiar A, Lucas M. Guidelines for the diagnosis and treatment of overactive bladder (OAB) and neurogenic detrusor overactivity (NDO). *Neurourol Urodyn*. 2014;33(suppl 3):S21–S25. doi:10.1002/nau.22631

10. Apostolidis A, Thompson C, Yan X, et al. An exploratory, placebo-controlled, dose-response study of the efficacy and safety of OnabotulinumtoxinA in spinal cord injury patients with urinary incontinence due to neurogenic detrusor overactivity. *World J Urol*. 2013;31(6):1469–1474. doi:10.1007/s00345-012-0984-0

11. Denys P, Del Popolo G, Amarenco G, et al. Efficacy and safety of two administration modes of an intra-detrusor injection of 750 units Dysport® (AbobotulinumtoxinA) in patients suffering from refractory neurogenic detrusor overactivity (NDO): a randomised placebo-controlled phase IIa study. *Neurourol Urodyn*. 2017;36(2):457–462. doi:10.1002/nau.22954

12. Hanno PM, Erickson D, Moldwin R, et al. Diagnosis and treatment of interstitial cystitis/bladder pain syndrome: AUA guideline amendment. *J Urol*. 2015;193(5):1545–1553. doi:10.1016/j.juro.2015.01.086

13. Moore DC, Cohn JA, Dmochowski RR. Use of botulinum toxin A in the treatment of lower urinary tract disorders: a review of the literature. *Toxins (Basel)*. 2016;8(4):88. doi:10.3390/toxins8040088

14. Amundsen CL, Richter HE, Menefee SA, et al. OnabotulinumtoxinA vs. sacral neuromodulation on refractory urgency urinary incontinence in women: a randomized clinical trial. *JAMA*. 2016;316(13):1366–1374. doi:10.1001/jama.2016.14617

15. Dowson C, Watkins J, Khan MS, et al. Repeated botulinum toxin type A injections for refractory overactive bladder: medium-term outcomes, safety profile, and discontinuation rates. *Eur Urol*. 2012;61(4):834–839. doi:10.1016/j.eururo.2011.12.011

16. Visco AG, Brubaker L, Richter HE, et al. Anticholinergic therapy vs. OnabotulinumtoxinA for urgency urinary incontinence. *N Engl J Med*. 2012;367(19):1803–1813. doi:10.1056/NEJMoa1208872

CHAPTER 20

Glabellar Rhytides

Background

The glabellar region occupies the area between the medial extent of the eyebrows and is formed by several muscles that function primarily for facial expressions. Vertical glabellar lines are formed from contraction of the corrugator muscles and horizontal lines by contraction of the procerus muscle. Several other muscles contribute to a lesser extent to the glabellar lines such as the depressor supercilii, nasalis, and orbicularis oculi muscles.[1] Treatment of the glabellar lines was the first FDA-approved cosmetic use for Onabotulinumtoxin A.[2]

Injection Technique and Dosing

Isolating the corrugator muscle between the thumb and index finger with the non-dominant hand allows for delineation of the muscle belly for injection. It is important to keep injections 1 cm above the orbital rim and to stay medial to the pupils. To inject procerus, ask the patient to furrow the eyebrows and inject midline into the belly of the muscle.

Injections should be performed intramuscularly into the muscle belly. Treatment should be individualized for location and dosage. The typical injection pattern involves two injections on each side for the corrugator muscles and a single central injection for the procerus muscle.[3] Men tend to have larger glabellar muscle mass than women and need a higher dose for effective control of the glabellar lines (Figure 20.1, Table 20.1).[3]

Complications

The most common side effect is bruising at the site of injection. Diplopia may occur if the botulinum toxin diffuses into the extraocular muscles. Ptosis may also occur if diffusion occurs into the levator palpebrae superioris muscle. If diplopia occurs, one may consider patching the eye for symptomatic relief. If ptosis

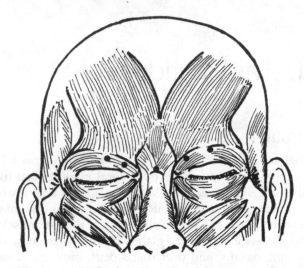

Figure 20.1 Injection localization for corrugator and procerus muscles.

Table 20.1 Suggested Dosing

	Botox®	Dysport®	Xeomin®	Myobloc®
Corrugator (total for both sides, divided between four sites)				
Author recommendations	Female 15–30 units	Female 30–90 units	Female 15–30 units	Female 2,000 units
	Male 20–40 units	Male 40–120 units	Male 20–40 units	Male 2,500 units
Per toxin package insert[4–6]	16 units†	40 units†	16 units†	—
Procerus (one site)				
Author recommendations	5–10 units	10–20 units	5–10 units	250–500 units
Per toxin package[4–6]	4 units†	10 units†	4 units†	—

†Denotes FDA-approved dosing.

occurs, it can be temporarily treated with apraclonidine 0.5% eye drops in the affected eye, up to four times daily as needed (off-label use). Diplopia or ptosis should typically self-resolve in 2 to 4 weeks.

Clinical Pearls and Pitfalls

- If the needle is inserted too superficially (subdermal), then it will be in the frontalis muscle.
- If the needle is injected too deep, then it will be in the periosteum, and can cause pain post-injection from inflammation of the periosteum.[7]

References

1. Frampton JE, Easthope SE. Botulinum toxin A (Botox® Cosmetic): a review of its use in the treatment of glabellar frown lines. *Am J Clin Dermatol*. 2003;4(10):709–725. doi:10.2165/00128071-200304100-00005
2. Dessy LA, Fallico N, Mazzocchi M, et al. Botulinum toxin for glabellar lines: a review of the efficacy and safety of currently available products. *Am J Clin Dermatol*. 2011;12(6):377–388. doi:10.2165/11592100-000000000-00000
3. Carruthers JD, Lowe NJ, Menter MA, Scuderi N. Double-blind, placebo-controlled study of the safety and efficacy of botulinum toxin type A for patients with glabellar lines. *Plast Reconstr Surg*. 2003;112(4):1089–1098. doi:10.1097/01.PRS.0000076504.79727.62
4. Allergan. Botox [package insert]. Published July 2020. https://media.allergan.com/actavis/actavis/media/allergan-pdf-documents/product-prescribing/20190620-BOTOX-100-and-200-Units-v3-0USPI1145-v2-0MG1145.pdf
5. Ipsen. Dysport [package insert]. Published September 2019. https://www.ipsen.com/websites/Ipsen_Online/wp-content/uploads/sites/9/2020/01/09195739/S115_2019_09_25_sBLA_Approval_PMR_Fulfilled_PI_MG_Sept-2019.pdf
6. Merz. Xeomin [package insert]. Published August 2020. https://dailymed.nlm.nih.gov/dailymed/fda/fdaDrugXsl.cfm?setid=ccdc3aae-6e2d-4cd0-a51c-8375bfee9458&type=display
7. Rappl T, Wurzer P, May S, et al. Three-dimensional evaluation of static and dynamic effects of botulinum toxin A on glabellar frown lines. *Aesthetic Plast Surg*. 2019;43(1):206–212. doi:10.1007/s00266-018-1230-y

Clinical Pearls and Pitfalls

- If the needle is inserted too superficially (subdermal), then it will be in the frontalis muscle.
- If the needle is inserted too deep, then it will be in the periosteum and can cause pain post-injection from inflammation of the periosteum.

References

1. [illegible] a review [illegible] glabellar [illegible] Dermatol. 2005;[illegible]
2. [illegible] review of the efficacy and safety of currently available products [illegible] Dermatol. 2011;[illegible]
3. Carruthers [illegible] double-blind, placebo-controlled [illegible] patients with [illegible] lines. [illegible] 2003;[illegible]
4. [illegible] media [illegible] product [illegible]
5. [illegible] 2019 [illegible] uploads/ [illegible] 2019 [illegible] Approval [illegible]
6. [illegible]
7. [illegible]

PART VI

Clinical Syndromes

CHAPTER 21

Neurogenic Thoracic Outlet Syndrome

Thoracic outlet syndrome (TOS) is defined as "upper extremity symptoms due to compression of the neurovascular bundle in the area of the neck just above the first rib."[1] The neurovascular bundle is compressed within the scalene triangle, which consists of the anterior and middle scalene muscles and the first rib.[2] Botulinum toxin has both diagnostic and therapeutic purposes. It may be used to provide temporary symptomatic relief and guide future decisions regarding surgical decompression.[2] When using botulinum toxin injections for neurogenic TOS, consider using smaller doses than listed in prior chapters, which are doses listed for hypertonicity. It is important to recognize that spread of the toxin to neighboring muscles can cause dysphagia and dysphonia.

Muscles to consider injecting for TOS are anterior scalene, middle scalene, ipsilateral trapezius, and pectoralis minor (Figure 21.1).

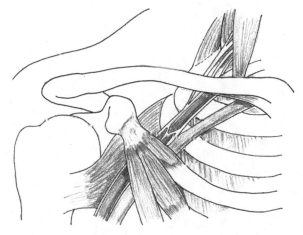

Figure 21.1 Thoracic outlet.

References

1. Sanders RJ, Hammond SL, Rao NM. Thoracic outlet syndrome: a review. *Neurologist*. 2008;14(6):365–373. doi:10.1097/NRL.0b013e318176b98d
2. Rahman A, Hamid A, Inozemtsev K, Nam A. Thoracic outlet syndrome treated with injecting botulinum toxin into middle scalene muscle and pectoral muscle interfascial planes: a case report. *A A Pract*. 2019;12(7): 235–237. doi:10.1213/XAA.0000000000000894

CHAPTER 22

Writer's Cramp

Writer's cramp is one of the most common focal limb dystonias. It presents as an involuntary, sustained posture or contraction of the hand, fingers, and/or arm muscles during writing. Writer's cramp can present in a flexion or extension pattern. Flexion pattern leads to increased pressure on the writing surface, bold script, and decreased ability to write in cursive. Extension pattern causes faint script, difficulty placing pen on paper, or difficulty holding the pen.[1] Muscle selection can be difficult due to the numerous muscles involved in the intricate and tightly coordinated task of writing.[2] Consider injecting only two to four key muscles initially and starting at a significantly lower dose than used for limb hypertonicity. Repeated treatments can be finessed with an increased number of muscles selected using smaller individual toxin doses. In general, treatment of flexion writer's cramp tends to need larger doses than extension writer's cramp.

Muscles to consider when evaluating writer's cramp (Figure 22.1):

- Flexor digitorum profundus
- Flexor carpi radialis
- Flexor digitorum superficialis
- Flexor carpi ulnaris
- Flexor pollicis longus
- Pronator teres
- Pronator quadratus
- Extensor digitorum
- Extensor carpi ulnaris
- Extensor pollicis longus
- Extensor pollicis brevis
- Extensor indicis
- . Adductor pollicis

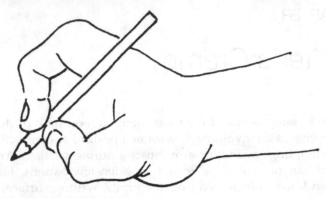

Figure 22.1 Flexion writer's cramp.

- Abductor digiti minimi
- Opponens pollicis
- Dorsal interosseous

References

1. Goldman JG. Writer's cramp. *Toxicon*. 2015;107(Pt A):98–104. doi:10.1016/j.toxicon.2015.09.024
2. Karp BI, Alter K. Muscle selection for focal limb dystonia. *Toxins (Basel)*. 2017;10(1):20. doi:10.3390/toxins10010020

CHAPTER 23

Hypertonicity Postures of Upper and Lower Limb

Spasticity is overactivity of muscles after injury to the central nervous system (CNS). When left untreated, it can lead to functional and medical complications.[1] Listed in the text that follows are common postures seen after injury to the CNS. These are some of the common muscles involved; however, not all muscles need to be injected simultaneously to get the desired outcome (Figures 23.1–23.14).

Common Postures of the Upper Extremity[1]

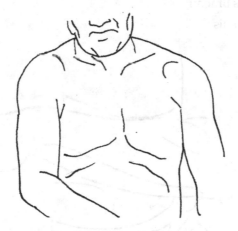

Figure 23.1 Adducted shoulder.

- Pectoralis major
- Pectoralis minor
- Latissimus dorsi

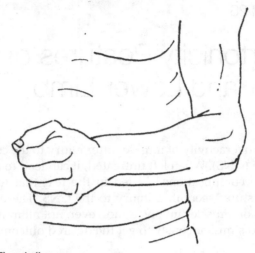

Figure 23.2 Flexed elbow.

- Brachioradialis
- Biceps brachii
- Brachialis

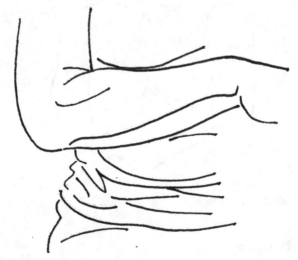

Figure 23.3 Pronated forearm.

- Pronator quadratus
- Pronator teres

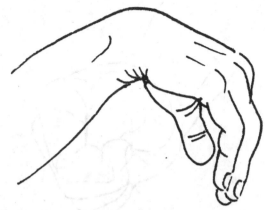

Figure 23.4 Flexed wrist.

- Flexor carpi radialis
- Flexor carpi ulnaris

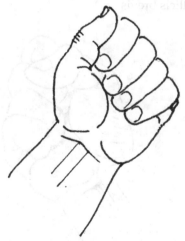

Figure 23.5 Flexed fingers.

- Flexor digitorum superficialis
- Flexor digitorum profundus

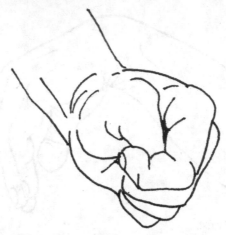

Figure 23.6 Thumb-in-palm.

- Flexor pollicis longus
- Adductor pollicis
- Flexor pollicis brevis

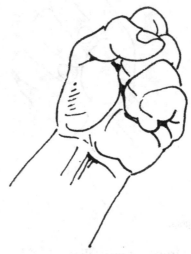

Figure 23.7 Clenched fist.

- Flexor digitorum superficialis
- Flexor digitorum profundus
- Flexor pollicis brevis
- Flexor pollicis longus
- Adductor pollicis longus

Common Postures of the Lower Extremity[2]

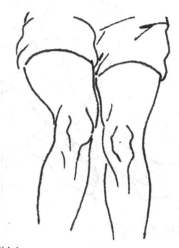

Figure 23.8 Adducted thigh.

- Adductor magnus
- Adductor longus
- Adductor brevis

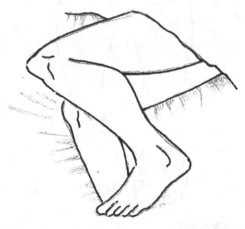

Figure 23.9 Flexed knee.

- Biceps femoris
- Semimembranosus
- Semitendinosus

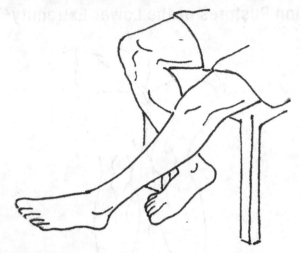

Figure 23.10 Extended knee.

- Rectus femoris
- Vastus lateralis
- Vastus medialis

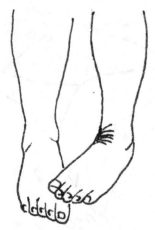

Figure 23.11 Equinovarus foot.

- Tibialis posterior
- Gastrocnemius
- Soleus

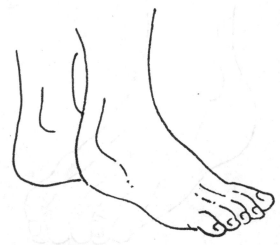

Figure 23.12 Plantar flexed foot.

- Gastrocnemius
- Soleus

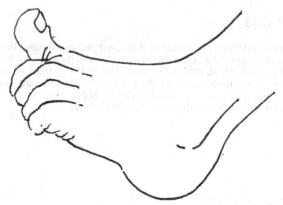

Figure 23.13 Striatal toe.

- Extensor hallucis longus

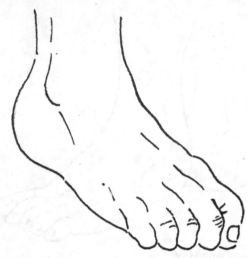

Figure 23.14 Flexed toes.

- Flexor digitorum longus
- Flexor digitorum brevis
- Flexor hallucis longus

References

1. Simpson DM, Patel AT, Alfaro A, et al. OnabotulinumtoxinA injection for poststroke upper-limb spasticity: guidance for early injectors from a Delphi Panel process. *PM R*. 2017;9(2):136–148. doi:10.1016/j.pmrj.2016.06.016
2. Esquenazi A, Alfaro A, Ayyoub Z, et al. OnabotulinumtoxinA for lower limb spasticity: guidance from a Delphi Panel approach. *PM R*. 2017;9(10):960–968. doi:10.1016/j.pmrj.2017.02.014

CHAPTER 24

Trigger Points

Background

Botulinum toxin has been used for treatment of many clinical disorders by producing skeletal muscle relaxation. The toxin inhibits the release of the neurotransmitter acetylcholine at the neuromuscular junction. In pain management, botulinum toxin has demonstrated an analgesic effect by reducing muscle hyperactivity.[1] The antinociceptive effect of botulinum toxin is attributed to blockage of pain transmitters such as substance P and glutamate.[2]

A myofascial trigger point (MTP) is defined as a palpable and hyperirritable nodule located in a taut band of muscle.[3] Myofascial pain syndromes (MPS) are most common between ages 27 to 50 years and in sedentary patients. Cervicothoracic and lumbosacral MPS are most common.

Despite the advances in clinical research, the exact pathophysiology of MPS is still unclear. Multiple studies have demonstrated that botulinum toxin injections into trigger points may alleviate pain; however, there is insufficient data to support its superiority over other treatments.

Injection Technique and Dosing

A myriad of injection techniques exist, and individual injector preference may vary. Trigger points are typically identified by a combination of palpation and patient report of pain (Figures 24.1 and 24.2). Once identified, a needle is inserted directly into the muscle at the trigger point at a 30° to 45° angle.

Dosing recommendations for injection of botulinum toxin into trigger points vary, but usually 5 to 10 units of Onabotulinumtoxin A or Incobotulinumtoxin A are injected per trigger point, with a total dose of 50 to 100 units depending on the number of injection sites and trigger points.[4]

If using Rimabotulinumtoxin B, then typically 500 to 1,000 units are injected per trigger point, for a total of 5,000 units.

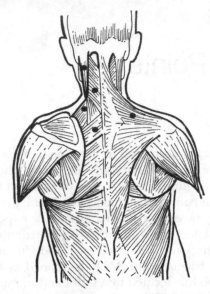

Figure 24.1 Common trigger point locations for posterior neck and upper back.

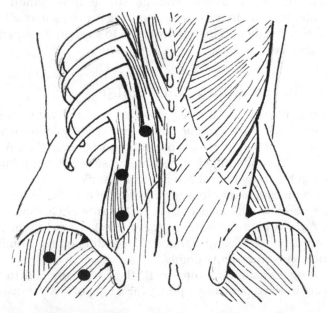

Figure 24.2 Common trigger point locations for posterior lower back.

Complications

The most common complications are pain, swelling, and bruising at the injection site.

Clinical Pearls and Pitfalls

- Deeper injections in the cervicothoracic area carry a risk of accidental pneumothorax.

References

1. Climent JM, Kuan T-S, Fenollosa P, Martin-del-Rosario F. Botulinum toxin for the treatment of myofascial pain syndromes involving the neck and back: a review from a clinical perspective. *Evid Based Complement Alternat Med*. 2013;2013:381459. doi:10.1155/2013/381459
2. Aoki KR. Evidence for antinociceptive activity of botulinum toxin type A in pain management. *Headache*. 2003;43(suppl 1):S9–S15. doi:10.1046/j.1526-4610.43.7s.3.x
3. Zhou JY, Wang D. An update on botulinum toxin A injections of trigger points for myofascial pain. *Curr Pain Headache Rep*. 2014;18(1):386. doi:10.1007/s11916-013-0386-z
4. Desai MJ, Shkolnikova T, Nava A, Inwald D. A critical appraisal of the evidence for botulinum toxin type A in the treatment for cervico-thoracic myofascial pain syndrome. *Pain Pract*. 2014;14(2):185–195. doi:10.1111/papr.12074

Suggested Readings

1) Royal College of Physicians, British Society of Rehabilitation Medicine, Chartered Society of Physiotherapy, Association of Chartered Physiotherapists in Neurology and the Royal College of Occupational Therapists. Spasticity in adults: management using botulinum toxin. National Guidelines. 2020. https://www.rcplondon.ac.uk/guidelines-policy/spasticityadults-management-using-botulinum-toxin

2) Jost W. *Pictorial Atlas of Botulinum Toxin Injection.* 2nd ed. Quintessence Publishing Co, Ltd; 2012.

3) Olver J, Esquenazi A, Fung VS, et al. Botulinum toxin assessment, intervention and aftercare for lower limb disorders of movement and muscle tone in adults: international consensus statement. *Eur J Neurol.* 2010;17(suppl 2):57–73. doi:10.1111/j.1468-1331.2010.03128.x

4) Sheean G, Lannin NA, Turner-Stokes L, et al. Botulinum toxin assessment, intervention and after-care for upper limb hypertonicity in adults: international consensus statement. *Eur J Neurol.* 2010;17(suppl 2):74–93. doi:10.1111/j.1468-1331.2010.03129.x

5) Perotto AO. *Anatomical Guide for the Electromyographer: The Limbs and Trunk.* 5th ed. Charles C Thomas Publisher, Ltd; 2011.

6) Jenkins DB. *Hollinshead's Functional Anatomy of the Limbs and Back.* 9th ed. Saunders Elsevier; 2009.

Index

Printed in the United States
by Baker & Taylor Publisher Services